Praise for
True Wellness for Your Heart

"Two healing traditions—East and West—are merged into this beautiful book about healing the heart. Clear, straightforward and well referenced, I recommend it to all who want to optimize their heart health."

—Wayne Jonas, MD, author, *How Healing Works*, executive director of Samueli Integrative Health Programs, clinical professor of Family Medicine Georgetown University, former director NIH Office of Alternative Medicine, former director World Health Organization Center for Traditional Medicine, former director of Medical Research Fellowship at Walter Reed Army Institute of Research.

"With a special focus on the prevention of cardiovascular disease, Drs. Catherine Kurosu and Aihan Kuhn bravely explore how practices of Western and Eastern medicine can coalesce to give rise to true wellness. In their innovative book, the authors weave two complementary threads that together are shaping the wellness revolution: technology-facilitated cutting-edge scientific advances, represented by biomedicine, and the human urge to reconnect with the inherent wisdom of the natural world, represented by traditional medical systems. An overview of the historical and philosophical roots, fundamental principles, trajectory of evolution, and scientific evidence for each system inform the potential clinical application of this integrated approach. Furthermore, the authors provide a roadmap for optimal health that includes a step-by-step guide for its implementation. Drs. Kurosu and Kuhn combine their knowledge and experience to empower patients in taking charge of their own health and encourage them to engage in shared decision making across cultural and paradigmatic borders. Their fundamental premise is that the combined knowledge and wisdom accumulated by humans all over the world and across time promises to effectively help us achieve true wellness."

—Rosa N. Schnyer, DAOM, IFMCP, L.Ac., Seeds of Wellness, doctor of Chinese medicine, licensed acupuncturist, assistant professor, certified functional medicine practitioner.

T0126188

"Bridging current knowledge of Western and Eastern medicine is no easy task. The authors have done an excellent job summarizing history and current understandings of both practices and manage to gracefully marry both. Being boarded in cardiology as well as acupuncture, I applaud the emphasis on lifestyle modification as well as the concise summary of cardiac ailments. A great read for both motivated patients and practitioners of Western as well as Eastern medicine."
—Bart G. Denys, MD, FACC, FSCAI

"A book about blending Eastern and Western medicine for heart health. In the newest book in their series, medical doctors Kuhn and Kurosu (*True Wellness: The Mind*, 2019, among others), who now practice holistic healing, examine cardiac health from an integrative perspective, combining Eastern and Western approaches to health care. As in their previous installments, the authors blend divergent tenets of Eastern and Western medicine—Kurosu trained in Canada and the United States, and Kuhn in China—into a cohesive wellness approach. They note some surprising parallels and highlight beneficial practices from each type of medicine and walk readers through ways to make them work together. This book specifically focuses on prevention and treatment of cardiac illnesses, combining traditional medicine with practices involving acupuncture, herbs, yoga, and qigong and rounding the regime out with tips on exercise, nutrition, meditation, and sleep. Their goal is educational, so the opening chapters aim to give readers a grounding in some of the science, history, and philosophy behind various treatments. They also include an in-depth examination of common cardiovascular problems, including hypertension, coronary artery disease, heart attacks, arrhythmias, and valve problems. Not all sections will apply to all readers, obviously, so some sections may be challenging to wade through. For instance, the book extensively details how blood vessels function, which sometimes requires the use of scientific language that casual readers may find difficult to grasp. However, the book also dispenses a good dose of general information about everyday lifestyle choices that are easy for anyone to comprehend and implement, and the authors liven up the concepts with examples from their own lives and practices. 'Homework,' including mental exercises as well as instructive diagrams and illustrations, will help readers customize their own wellness plans. The authors support their advice with exhaustive citations, which makes the book feel more comprehensive than other similar works.

A detailed and appealing work on wellness."

—KIRKUS Reviews

"This book combines Eastern and Western medical modalities for our well-being—in particular, our cardiovascular system. On top of writing an informative, easy-to-comprehend text, the authors have accomplished a unique feat by applying the concept of the whole system (our body and environment) to tackle the many and complicated cardiovascular issues that pervade populations today. I consider this book a guideline for our well-being and cardiovascular health. If one can follow the authors' recommendations with consistent practice, as outlined in the book, one will surely experience a better quality of life, not to mention increased productivity in all areas. If we all would do the same, we could drastically reduce our overall cost of health care. Thus, I recommend that every family get at least one copy of this book and reward yourself with healthier well-being. Preventative care is the best health care!"

—H. Bill Xie, MD, PhD

"*True Wellness for Your Heart* is the perfect book for those interested in the comparative histories, philosophies and applications of Eastern and Western medicine. More importantly, it provides a compelling argument against the pervasive notion that these disciplines are mutually exclusive philosophies, and provides a step-by-step evidence-based guide on the integration of these philosophies for optimal health and wellness. I particularly appreciated the actionable, practical tips to help put knowledge into practice. As a primary care physician, I highly recommend this book to colleagues and patients alike."

—Kimberly Rogers, MD, Diplomate American Board of Lifestyle Medicine

"This book will help readers understand how the combination of Western (modern) and Eastern medicine could promote people's health and how this combination could benefit people's well-being. Eastern (Chinese) medicine is not only treating diseases, but also using some good modalities to prevent illness or reduce the possibility of diseases. I believe practicing qigong and other movements mentioned in this book are effective methods for making your cardiovascular system healthier and reducing occurrences of cardiovascular diseases. Herbal medicine and acupuncture are excellent alternative for people suffering from these diseases. In addition, these authors are experienced physicians in both Western and Eastern (Chinese) medicine, which is helpful for providing a deeper view of both medical systems."

—Sherry Zhou, MD, endocrinologist

"*True Wellness for Your Heart* is such a refreshing book. In this book, Drs. Kurosu and Kuhn focus on the whole person, incorporating Western and Eastern medicine, free of pharmaceutical or political bias. This book will benefit not only care providers but also anyone who has a pumping heart. Those who have cardiovascular diseases, hypertension, hyperlipidemia, or coronary artery disease or heart attacks will definitely find helpful tips in this book, but my hope would be that people would read this book *before* they manifest heart problems and incorporate the suggested therapeutic modalities in their life to *prevent* heart issues. Keep a strong pumping heart!"

—Katsuya Andrew Iizuka, MD, family medicine, Hawai'i Pacific Health

"As a practicing attorney and family court judge in Hawai'i for more than forty-five years, I have seen the intersection of health and wellness—both physical and mental health—affect individuals and their immediate and extended families from young children through grandparents. As much as we might wish a pill or surgery to be the instant cure for all that ails us, it is not to be. Drs. Kurosu and Kuhn are well versed in Western and Eastern medicine and combine those approaches to focus us on tending to our whole being. Their medical description of how our heart and circulatory system works is written in language the layman can understand. The combination with Eastern perspectives about the workings of mind and body make sense even to a linear thinker.

I understand that there are more volumes of *True Wellness* focusing on additional health issues. I look forward to reading those as well and incorporating the doctors' suggestions into my daily routine."

—Judge Karen M. Radius (Ret.)

CATHERINE KUROSU, MD, LAc
AIHAN KUHN, CMD, OBT

TRUE WELLNESS FOR YOUR HEART

Combine the best of
Western and Eastern medicine for
optimal heart health

YMAA Publication Center
Wolfeboro, New Hampshire

YMAA Publication Center, Inc.
PO Box 480
Wolfeboro, New Hampshire 03894
1-800-669-8892 • info@ymaa.com • www.ymaa.com

ISBN: 9781594397356 (print) • ISBN: 9781594397363 (ebook)

10 9 8 7 6 5 4 3 2 1

Publisher's Cataloging in Publication
Names: Kurosu, Catherine, author. | Kuhn, Aihan, author.
Title: True wellness for your heart : combine the best of Western and Eastern
    medicine for optimal heart health / Catherine Kurosu, Aihan Kuhn.
Description: Wolfeboro, New Hampshire : YMAA Publication Center, Inc., [2020] |
    Series: True wellness | Includes bibliographical references and index.
Identifiers: ISBN: 9781594397356 (print) | 9781594397363 (ebook) |
    LCCN: 2020931874
Subjects: LCSH: Cardiovascular system—Diseases—Prevention. | Cardiovascular
    system—Diseases—Treatment. | Coronary heart disease—Prevention. | Coronary
    heart disease—Treatment. | Heart—Diseases—Prevention. | Heart—Diseases—
    Treatment. | Hypertension—Prevention. | Myocardial infarction—Prevention. |
    Arrhythmia—Prevention. | Energy medicine. | Holistic medicine. | Medicine,
    Chinese. | Self-care, Health. | Alternative medicine. | Health—Alternative
    treatment. | Health behavior. | Qi gong—Therapeutic use. | Mind and body. |
    Well-being. | BISAC: MEDICAL / Preventive medicine. | HEALTH & FITNESS /
    Diseases / Heart. | HEALTH & FITNESS / Healthy Living.
Classification: LCC: RC685.C6 K87 2020 | DDC: 616.1/2305—dc23

NOTE TO READERS

The practices, treatments, and methods described in this book should not be used as an alternative to professional medical diagnosis or treatment. The authors and publisher of this book are NOT RESPONSIBLE in any manner whatsoever for any injury or negative effects that may occur through following the instructions and advice contained herein.

It is recommended that before beginning any treatment or exercise program, you consult your medical professional to determine whether you should undertake this course of practice.

Printed in Canada

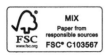

Table of Contents

Books in the True Wellness series
True Wellness
True Wellness: The Mind
True Wellness for Your Heart
True Wellness for Your Gut

Also by Aihan Kuhn
Natural Healing with Qigong
Simple Chinese Medicine
Tai Chi in 10 Weeks

Dedicated to my family—
Gerry Kuhn, Sharon Kuhn, and Peter Kuhn

For Michael M. Zanoni—
Teacher, Colleague, Friend

Foreword

HEART DISEASE REMAINS the number one cause of death in the western world in men as well as women and is rapidly catching up in developing countries. Despite significant progress in medication and available therapies in cardiology, the human cost and financial burden remain high.

True Wellness for Your Heart is a refreshing and successful approach to integrating Western and Eastern medical concepts. The authors provide a concise history of the evolution of cardiac knowledge and understanding from both sides. It is indeed remarkable how closely East and West parallel their approach to the treatment of cardiovascular disease, emphasizing lifestyle and wellness.

This book is a must read for patients who want to learn more about their disease process and available therapeutic options. It is equally instructive for both Eastern and Western medical practitioners who want to offer their patients an expanded range of therapeutic modalities. The authors encourage patients to learn about their options and suggest constructive ways to gracefully discuss with their practitioner. Finally, the lifestyle modification instructions are universal, well presented, and well worth the cost of admission.

Bart G. Denys, M.D.
Fellow of the American College of Cardiology
Fellow of the American Society of Cardiovascular
Angiography and Interventions
Fellow of the American Academy of Medical Acupuncture

Preface

THE HEART IS A PUMP.

And yet, it is so much more than that. Through the ages, countless works of art have been centered on the affairs of the heart: not the mechanical pump that pushes blood through our vessels to nourish our bodies, but rather, the emotional heart that nourishes our souls. Thousands of poems, songs, plays, novels, paintings, statues, and movies have been devoted to the attributes of the heart. These include love, loyalty, courage, and honesty.

Even modern heart specialists, such as famed cardiovascular surgeon Dr. Mehmet Oz and renowned interventional cardiologists Dr. Mimi Guarneri, Dr. Sandeep Jauhar, and Dr. Kavitha Chinnaiyan, acknowledge that a mechanistic approach to treating heart disease is insufficient. They have all written persuasively about the role that emotional, physical, and spiritual health plays in the healing and even prevention of cardiovascular disease. These physicians, and many more, assert that a reductionist medical model that searches for a single cause for a given heart condition will miss the complex interplay of factors that influence cardiovascular health. Such factors are unique to each person: from genetic predisposition, home environment, and life experiences to socioeconomic status, environmental pollution, and geopolitical issues. These factors affect the body, mind, and spirit and influence all aspects of heart health.

As individuals, we may feel overwhelmed as we strive to change our internal and external environments to promote healing. Large changes in behavior are difficult to implement and maintain, but more and more research is showing that smaller changes in lifestyle choices create internal resilience to external factors that may be beyond our control.

The origins of disease are highly complex, especially with respect to the chronic diseases of Western societies, such as heart disease, type 2 diabetes, autoimmune conditions, and some gastrointestinal disorders. For many of these conditions, the biomedical model may not be the best way to institute effective health care. A growing body of evidence suggests that optimizing the way we eat, move, think, and sleep can do more to reverse chronic illness than medications or surgery. Adopting such lifestyle changes may even help to prevent these conditions in the first place.

The importance of the idea that what we eat and our levels of activity, sleep quality, and calmness of mind influence our health is not a new concept in medicine at all. In Western medicine, the importance of these factors was considered vital millennia ago and is reemerging today. Increasingly, students of Western biomedicine are being trained to consider all aspects of an individual and their illness. This patient-centered model is called "biopsychosocial medicine." Practitioners who hold this viewpoint evaluate not just the biological cause of a disease but also the psychological, emotional, spiritual, and socioeconomic factors involved. All these elements can both affect and be affected by the disease process. Through this understanding, more and more medical practitioners are able to help patients heal and maintain optimal health.

Our purpose in writing *True Wellness for Your Heart* is to educate readers about how the heart and blood vessels work and how their daily choices can positively influence their cardiovascular health. It is not enough to simply take whatever medication your doctor prescribes. You can be an active participant in your own revitalization, whether you are recovering from heart disease or wish to prevent it. Your decisions about sleep, food, restorative practices, exercise, relationships, and community all affect your heart. Our hope is that you will use this book as a guide to enhance not only your cardiovascular health but also your complete well-being.

We wish you every success on your journey.

Aihan Kuhn, CMD, OBT
Catherine Kurosu, MD, LAc

CHAPTER 1

The Cardiovascular System, Health, and Healing, from an East/ West Perspective

A Brief History of the Heart

The heart and its workings are still incompletely understood. Certainly, the mechanical aspects of the heart are well documented. But, the emotional heart and the heart-mind connection still present an enigma. We intuitively know that our feelings can affect our cardiac physiology. Even our everyday language supports the notion that the heart is intimately involved in our emotional life. When we are discouraged, we say we are "disheartened"; when grief-stricken, we are "broken-hearted." We call people "warm-hearted" or "cold-hearted" depending on our perception of their ability to be empathetic. If we think someone is overly sensitive, we say that they take things "too much to heart." We linguistically tie the heart to not only our feelings but also to our thinking mind. Actors and musicians the world over learn their parts "by heart." When we change our opinion, we have a "change of heart." When we "get to the heart of the matter," we use our intellect to decipher a problem to its essential indivisible root.

Affairs of the heart can have very physical consequences. We know that our bodies perceive heightened emotions such as grief and fear as reaction to a physical threat. In such a situation, our hearts beat faster and our blood pressure rises as the body prepares to either fight or flee. This automatic response, when overstimulated, can damage the heart muscle, the blood vessels, and the small arteries that nourish the heart itself. The fight-or-flight response occurs during periods of psychological stress, even if there is no actual physical danger. During the last century, numerous observational studies have shown that it is possible to die from stressors such as a broken heart or overwhelming emotional strain.[1] In the following chapters, we discuss the physiology of the heart and blood vessels and how our biopsychosocial state influences our cardiovascular health; but for the moment, let's look at how our understanding of the heart has evolved over millennia and across hemispheres.

The heart remained a mystery in both the East and the West for centuries. Although the heart was described as the body's emotional and spiritual center by many ancient societies, its exact function was not entirely known. This was due, in part, to prohibition against human dissection in some societies, such as India.

The ancient Egyptians had a remarkably accurate understanding of the heart and the circulatory system. In the late nineteenth century, a German Egyptologist named Georg Moritz Ebers acquired a compilation of Egyptian medical texts dating from approximately 1550 BCE. This document, known as the Ebers Papyrus, contains seven hundred remedies and incantations, along with a description of the circulatory system that correctly placed the heart at the center of blood supply, stating that the blood vessels connected the heart to the major organs. As we will see, this schema was still incomplete.

In ancient Greece, the birthplace of Western medicine, the physician Hippocrates (460–360 BCE) notated very precise symptoms of heart disease, though the exact mechanism and anatomy were not entirely understood. The philosopher Aristotle (384–322 BCE) had a strong background in medicine because his father was a physician. Around the time of Hippocrates and Aristotle there was considerable controversy about the true nature of the heart. Some doctors felt that the heart was

---

1. Sandeep Jauhar, *Heart* (New York: Farrar, Straus, and Giroux, 2018), 23–31.

the seat of the intellect, whereas others argued that the intellect was housed in the brain. Hippocrates declared that consciousness and intellect rested in the brain,[2] but Aristotle supported the notion that human intelligence, movement, and the physical heat of the body emanated from the heart. He described the other organs such as the lungs and the brain as supporting players, whose sole purpose was to cool the heart and prevent it from overheating.[3]

The Chinese of the same era recognized that the heart regulated the flow of blood, but they also felt that the heart housed the spirit. The Heart Spirit was responsible for the connection of the individual with others in the family and society. Furthermore, the healthy Heart Spirit would ensure that this connection manifested at the right time and space with appropriate behavior and speech.[4]

In Europe, the Roman physician Galen (130–210 CE) performed surgeries on wounded gladiators and dissections on various animals. Based on his observations, he devised a theory of human circulation that stated the liver turned food into blood. The blood was then drawn into the heart, where it moved from the right side of the heart to the left side through invisible pores. While on the left side of the heart, the blood was mixed with "vital spirits." The left heart created heat to move the blood to the rest of the body in a unidirectional manner, where it was consumed entirely. He also proposed that the heart was nourished by blood left inside its chambers and that the pulse that could be felt at various points on the body was the result of inherent contractility of the blood vessel in question.

Galen's theories of human circulation held sway in Europe from the third to seventeenth centuries; however, in thirteenth-century Persia, a physician named Ibn al-Nafis took issue with many of Galen's assertions.

---

2. Arnold M. Katz and Phyllis B. Katz, "Disease of the Heart in the Works of Hippocrates," *British Heart Journal*, May 1, 1962, http://dx.doi.org/10.1136/hrt.24.3.257, https://heart.bmj.com/content/heartjnl/24/3/257.full.pdf.

3. Stanford University, "A History of the Heart," https://web.stanford.edu/class/history13/earlysciencelab/body/heartpages/heart.html, accessed January 3, 2019.

4. Ted Kaptchuk, *The Web That Has No Weaver* (New York: McGraw-Hill, 2000), 88.

In his *Commentary on Anatomy,* written in 1242, Ibn al-Nafis correctly stated that the heart received its nourishment from the coronary arteries, that the pulse was a reflection of the force of the heart's contraction, and that there were no invisible pores between the right and left sides of the heart. Unfortunately, this commentary was not known in Europe and was almost lost to antiquity until a copy was rediscovered in 1924.[5]

Other men of science who contributed to the understanding of the human heart were Leonardo da Vinci (1452–1519) and Andreas Vesalius (1514–1564). Leonardo correctly described the turbulence of blood flow responsible for the closing of the valves that separated the chambers of the heart and blood vessels. He also noted the thickening of arteries that we now know as atherosclerotic plaque. Vesalius corrected some of Galen's errors, particularly the idea that there were invisible pores within the heart. Vesalius correctly theorized that in order for blood to get from the right side of the heart to the left, it had to pass through the lungs. Vesalius did not realize all of Galen's mistakes, however. He still promoted the idea that the liver created the blood, which was then totally used up by the body.[6] Not until the next century was this error put to rest.

In 1628, the English anatomist William Harvey published his monograph, *De motu cordis,* in which he described a series of experiments that led him to correctly conclude that the heart was a pump that circulated blood through a closed circuit. By calculating how much blood the heart would pump out with each beat, and noting that the heart beat approximately seventy-two times per minute, Harvey showed that it would be impossible for the liver to create enough blood to keep a person alive if it were completely consumed. By his calculations, the liver would need to manufacture five hundred pounds of blood each hour. Harvey correctly surmised that blood keeps circulating and carried something within it that would nourish the body. The blood transported the nourishment, but was not itself consumed. In spite of the fact that

---

5. Sandeep Jauhar, *Heart* (New York: Farrar, Straus, and Giroux, 2018), 41.
6. Jauhar, *Heart*, 42–43.

Harvey knew that blood traveled through the lungs, he was unaware of the fact that oxygen was transferred from the lungs to cells within the blood. These discoveries were made in the eighteenth century.[7]

Dr. Sandeep Jauhar, in his excellent book, *Heart: A History*, takes an in-depth look at the development of modern cardiology and cardiovascular surgery. It is a fascinating journey, seeing how this field transformed medicine by treating conditions that would once carry the certainty of premature demise. Yet even now, in the twenty-first century, when modern miracles such as open-heart surgery and transplantation are commonplace, we are still struggling to control rampant cardiovascular disease—the number one cause of death worldwide. We have a good understanding of the mechanics of the heart, but an incomplete comprehension of the myriad biopsychosocial influences on cardiovascular health. Why is sleep so important for heart health? Why does depression increase the risk of high blood pressure? Does loneliness cause heart attacks? Can a person really die from a broken heart?

In his fascinating book, *How Healing Works*, Dr. Wayne Jonas recounts the amazing finding that rabbits who were cuddled and played with daily had 60 percent less plaque in their arteries than rabbits who were ignored, in spite of the fact that both groups were fed large amounts of fat and had elevated cholesterol levels.[8] Is it possible that love, attention, and caring can create resilience to heart disease?

Modern medicine is looking closely at all these questions and many more. For example, why do members of certain communities have fewer heart attacks? Around the world, in the East and the West, there are societies in which heart disease is virtually unheard of. You might be interested in learning from these people about how to decrease your risk of heart disease. How can you modify not only your diet and exercise habits but also your emotional well-being, to live a healthy and happy life?

---

7. Jauhar, *Heart*, 45–46.

8. Wayne Jonas, *How Healing Works* (New York: Penguin Random House, 2018), 145.

As we stated in our first book, *True Wellness*, we firmly believe the answers to these questions lie in the integration of the cutting-edge science of the West and the ancient wisdom of the East. To understand how these modalities can be dovetailed, we would like to present the next two sections from that work and undertake a short discussion of the history and philosophy of both systems. We will also discuss the science behind the Eastern healing arts and how your Western health-care provider can incorporate Eastern medicine into your care. Once this groundwork has been laid, we will start to answer all these heart-related questions and help you develop strategies to minimize your risk of cardiovascular disease.

The History and Philosophy of Western Medicine

Hippocrates is considered the father of Western medicine. He felt that a clear understanding of the patient's way of life and constitution was essential in order to provide appropriate medical care. He particularly emphasized balance in daily living regarding food and exercise. In ancient Greece, the human body was thought to be composed of material substances called "humors": blood, water, and bile. Additionally, the humors were associated with certain qualities (hot, cold, moist, and dry) and elements (earth, air, fire, and water). Perfect health was considered to be the ideal equilibrium of the humors, qualities, and elements within each individual, and disease was the result of imbalances among these components.

Even prior to the birth of Hippocrates, Greek philosophers and physicians were fascinated with the natural world and, like the Chinese, used observations of their environment to explain human growth and development. It was thought that the universe consisted of pairs of opposite qualities, such as hot and cold, moist and dry. Harmony between these pairs was considered paramount, as an imbalance could result in disease. This principle of paired opposites is also seen in the Chinese theory of yin and yang, which we discuss shortly.

Another parallel between Eastern and Western medical thought was the concept of "vitalism." This is the notion that, within the human body, an active and intelligent force instinctively maintains the health of the whole person. This "vital force" is similar to the Chinese concept of qi.

This idea of a dynamic energy within every individual was central to the art and science of medicine in Europe until after the Renaissance, during the Scientific Revolution (1450–1630 CE). During the Scientific Revolution, doctors were able to use advancing technology to examine the intricate workings of the human body and their environment. For example, in 1609, the light microscope was invented and, for the first time, doctors and scientists could see organisms that were invisible to the naked eye. They called such organisms microbes. Over the next two centuries, into the 1800s, an understanding of these organisms developed. It was proven that microbes, further classified as bacteria, viruses, and molds, could cause disease. Once it was known that specific organisms caused specific diseases, treatments were created that could cure many illnesses that had previously resulted in severe disability or death. Over time, vaccines were invented that could prevent some diseases altogether. The study of microbiology and the development of antibiotics and vaccines are some of the most significant discoveries of Western medicine.

With this astounding success in the treatment of infectious disease, Western physicians realized that if they could find the cause of an illness, they might be able to develop a cure. From this point onward, the study of medicine focused on the search for the simplest single explanation for the origin of a whole host of ailments. By this time, the Industrial Revolution in Europe was in full swing, and the study of medicine was influenced greatly by the societal changes of this era. Factories emerged, and every part of the production process was compartmentalized. No longer did an artisan see the creation of an item through from start to finish. Rather, a worker manufactured one portion of the item, then passed it on to the next worker and then the next, until completion. This fragmentation became pervasive in Western medicine. Technology gave physicians and scientists the ability to break down biochemical and physiological processes into ever-smaller component parts; this has led to an unprecedented understanding of the complexity of the human body.

New discoveries are still being made: from the understanding that a person's constitution can be passed down to offspring to the complete mapping of the human genome, and from realizing that living things are made up of cells to understanding how these cells function and how we can use modern medicine to change these processes. New drugs, new surgical techniques, and new therapies are continually being discovered, trialed, and then, if successful, offered to patients. One of the main difficulties of this explosion of knowledge is how to master it and implement it correctly. The production line increased efficiency during the Industrial Revolution, with each worker perfecting a certain aspect in the manufacturing process. Modern medicine has also undergone a similar division of labor.

With the increasing complexity of biomedicine, it has become impossible to know everything about the human body, how we get sick, how we heal, and all the possible therapeutic interventions that can be used for every possible illness. Medical students the world over gain basic knowledge in anatomy, physiology, and biochemistry, then branch out to learn about the many causes of disease and how to cure or improve a patient's condition. Upon graduating from medical school, young doctors in most countries are required to train further. They choose from many branches of medicine and become specialists in that field. Even those doctors who want to become family physicians do a three-year residency in general medicine to hone their skills. Others choose among general surgery, internal medicine, obstetrics and gynecology, psychiatry, radiology, or pathology. After completing at least four years in their specialty, they can then subspecialize—they can focus on the medical or surgical aspects of any single body part or process. From the brain to the feet and everything in between, you can find a subspecialist to meet your needs.

But, even as a subspecialist, it is difficult to keep up with every new scientific discovery in the field. Subdividing and specializing medical research and care is a way of trying to achieve this impossible task. Similarly, the search for the single underlying cause of a particular disease is a way for modern medicine to develop treatments that hope to correct problems at the cellular, genetic, or molecular level of the body. In many instances, this approach has been spectacularly successful. For example, the discovery of the underlying cause of type 1 diabetes led to the discovery of insulin and methods for isolating it from animal sources. We are now able to manufacture insulin synthetically. Furthermore, we can even transplant the cells that create insulin, allowing diabetics to survive. Without the curiosity and ingenuity of physicians and scientists, this and other medical breakthroughs would not exist.

For many conditions, however, this reductionist approach has not been successful or has even created more problems. The biomedical model of seeking out a solitary cause for an illness may overlook the possibility of interplay among many factors that can contribute to a disease. These factors can be specific to an individual, like genetics, family environment, and personal life experience, or they can be factors that affect the community at large, like environmental pollution, food additives, and poor access to markets with fresh produce or green spaces in which to exercise.

The dynamics of the origins of disease are highly complex, especially with respect to the chronic diseases of Western societies, such as heart disease, type 2 diabetes, autoimmune conditions, and some gastrointestinal disorders. For many of these conditions, the biomedical model may not be the best way to institute effective health care. A growing body of evidence suggests that optimizing the way we eat, move, think, and sleep can do more to reverse chronic illness than medications or surgery. Adopting such lifestyle changes may even help to prevent these conditions in the first place.

With the realization that so many of our modern day illnesses stem from being sleep-deprived, over-fed, under-exercised, and stressed, the philosophy of Western medicine is coming full circle. We are returning to the idea that physicians must consider all aspects of a person and that person's illness, just as Hippocrates did. In this patient-centered model, the emotional, spiritual, psychological, and socioeconomic factors involved are examined alongside the physical aspects of a disease.

This understanding, rooted in the origins of Western medicine, can help medical providers guide patients toward optimal health and healing.

The History and Philosophy of Eastern Medicine

Before discussing the chronology of Eastern medicine, an appreciation of its philosophy is extremely important. The principles of Eastern medicine hinge on the concept that man is inseparable from the universe. This notion comes from the observations and practices of Daoism. Daoism is a philosophical system that was reportedly founded by Laozi (b. 604 BCE). Although Laozi formulated the tenets of Daoism, it was his students and followers who wrote the majority of the formal texts that are the foundation of this philosophy. Prior to the advent of Daoism in China, as in every primitive civilization, the ancients observed the changes that took place over time in the world around them. They noted the cycles of the moon, planets, and stars. These celestial patterns were correlated with weather changes, growing seasons, and animal migrations. Daoism grew out of this naturalist school of thought as it attempted to understand man's place in the order of the universe. This law of nature is called the Dao. In English, this translates as "the Way" or "the Path." The Dao represents the basic principles from which all phenomena follow, including all aspects of human behavior.

In addition to the ideas of the Dao and the phases in the physical world that change over time, Daoist thinkers helped formalize the concept of the unity of opposites within nature. This is the basis of yin-yang theory, for which Eastern medicine is known. By starting with the concept of opposition to describe the relationship between two entities, Daoists formulated a dynamic view of the world that could be used to explain universal processes. A classic example of this mode of thought is the observation that there is always a sunny side and a shady side to a hill. Labels are given to each item being described, as either yin or yang, depending on its degree of substantiality. If something is more passive and receptive in nature, it is yin. If it is more active and dynamic, it is yang. But these definitions have meaning only when compared one to the other. Any of the pairs that embody yin and yang cannot be separated and are not absolute.

The yin-yang experience is a fundamental factor in the development of the Daoist metaphysic. Far from designating yang as "something" and yin as "nothing," Daoism recognizes that both are active and that one creates the other.[9] For example, the ceramic of a teacup would be considered yang and the space within the teacup considered yin. It is the space that is filled, and therefore makes the ceramic useful as a teacup. The yin and the yang of the cup are inseparable.

From this thought arises the realization that the part and the whole must exist simultaneously. The infinite exists at every singular point in space, and eternity is found in every individual moment. The Daoist consideration of the infinite and the yin-yang experience infuse themselves into the practice of Eastern medicine by virtue of the fact that dysfunction within the patient, known as the pattern of disharmony, cannot be viewed separately from the patient herself. The part and whole exist together and define each other.

In addition to the concepts of Dao and yin-yang, the recognition of the phases of the universe was developed into the theory known as Wu Xing, or Five Phases. Wu Xing has also been translated as Five Elements; however, many scholars state that this characterization is incorrect. The word "element" implies a component part or constituent ingredient; the word "phase" denotes a dynamic process. In his iconic book, *The Web That Has No Weaver*, Dr. Ted Kaptchuk describes the Five Phases as patterns that occur in dynamic systems. Each phase has a designated name and displays a set of particular characteristics.[10] The phases are known as Wood, Fire, Earth, Metal, and Water. The names of the phases are not as important as each set of characteristic qualities and functions. Wood represents growth. Fire represents maximal growth that

---

9. Michael M. Zanoni, PhD, conversation with author (CK), April 10, 2011.

10. Ted J. Kaptchuk, *The Web That Has No Weaver* (New York: McGraw Hill, 2000), 437.

has reached its apex and will plateau or decline. Metal is emblematic of decline. Water denotes a profound state of rest that has reached its nadir and will shift toward growth or activity. Earth represents balance.[11] If you imagine a pendulum swinging to and fro, the Earth Phase would be the moment at which the pendulum is hanging straight down. The patterns of the Five Phases can be seen in the ebb and flow of all natural and even man-made phenomena: human growth, maturation, and decline; the changing of the seasons; economic expansion and recession; the rise and fall of political powers. In both Eastern and Western medicine, the functional systems of the body experience this ebb and flow as constant self-regulation to maintain balance and optimize metabolic processes. In the following diagram of the Five Phases, the terms "generate" and "control" describe appropriate self-regulation between the functional systems, whereas the term "insult" describes a situation in which a functional system is overactive due to lack of control by another system. This creates abnormal symptoms in both areas of influence.

Diagram of the Five Phases

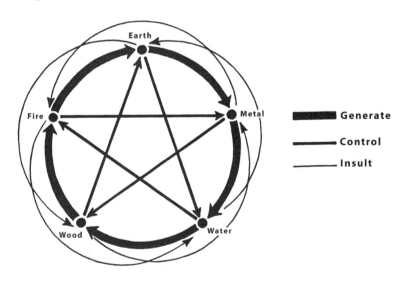

---

11. Kaptchuk, *Web That Has No Weaver*, 438.

As long ago as the fourth century BCE, the Five Phases construct was used to understand and interrelate naturally occurring events. This understanding was applied to medicine as well as other disciplines, including astrology, social politics, and natural sciences.[12] Using this paradigm, Daoist physicians looked at the human body as a microcosm of the universe and sought to use the natural laws of the universe to maintain a harmonious balance. They acknowledged that this balance must occur internally and also with the patient's external environment. Following the principles of Daoism, which emphasize moderation and equilibrium, the patient would be cautioned to follow the middle path in all aspects of life: to rest but also exercise, to work but have time for leisure, to eat a variety of healthy foods but neither too much nor too little. By achieving this equilibrium, the movement of the intelligent vital force within the body (called qi) would be smooth. This free movement of qi would maintain optimal health.

In 1973, in the Chinese province of Hunan, a famous archeological dig discovered silk texts that discussed subjects as diverse as astrology, art, military strategy, philosophy, and medicine. There were even two copies of Laozi's *Dao De Ching* found in the Mawangdui tombs (King Ma's Mound). Scientific methods were used to date the texts from approximately 200 BCE, and the tomb itself had been sealed in 168 BCE. The medical texts cover physiology, illness, surgery, herbal treatments, and what has been translated as "macrobiotic hygiene." Macrobiotic hygiene involves not only the body but also the spirit; this section discusses longevity, sexuality, and diet. Breathing and physical exercises are recommended for treating illness and cultivating health, and there are also writings on magic and incantations.[13]

Illness is described in the Mawangdui medical manuscripts as being the result of a disturbance in the movement of qi within the eleven

---

12. Joseph Helms, *Acupuncture Energetics: A Clinical Approach for Physicians* (Berkeley, CA: Medical Acupuncture Publishers, 1995), 17.

13. Donald J. Harper, *Early Chinese Medical Literature: The Mawangdui Medical Manuscripts* (London: Routledge, Taylor, and Francis, 1998), 6.

vessels of the body. These vessels that contain qi are different from the arteries and veins that contain blood. The treatment advocated at the time involved cauterization of the qi vessels. There is no mention of using acupuncture needles to correct the flow of qi. Instead, the medical practitioners who wrote these manuscripts advocated the use of food, herbs, breath control, and exercise to improve the flow of qi and achieve a long and vibrant life.

This approach to good health was formalized in the classic medical text of the Han dynasty (206 BCE–220 CE), the *Huang Di Nei Jing* (*The Yellow Emperor's Classic of Internal Medicine*). It is thought that this text is a compilation of medical writings from practitioners of earlier centuries, which takes the form of a discussion between the Yellow Emperor (Huang Di) and his minister; it is significant in that it was the first known text to move away from shamanism and supernatural causes of disease. Like the Mawangdui medical manuscripts, the *Huang Di Nei Jing* discusses the prevention and treatment of illness through diet, exercise, and herbs. Acupuncture theory is well described in the second volume of this text. The principles of energy flow within the body (qi), yin-yang theory, and diagnostic techniques are also discussed.

Around the first century BCE, the art of acupuncture using metal needles was formalized. Some researchers of Chinese medical history state that acupuncture arose from the practice of using sharpened stones and bones to lance infected skin, allowing the body to heal. However, scholars such as Paul Unschuld and Donald Harper state that the vessel theory and treatment paradigm delineated in the Mawangdui medical manuscripts was the necessary precursor to acupuncture theory as described in the *Huang Di Nei Jing*.[14]

Through trial and error, the Chinese determined that placing acupuncture needles at specific sites would give consistent and reproducible results. By the time the *Huang Di Nei Jing* was written, the intricate system of acupuncture points and qi flow within acupuncture channels was well established. Twelve paired principal channels, or vessels, were

---

14. Harper, *Early Chinese Medical Literature*, 5.

The Body Channels

Two Centerline Channels
Conception Vessel (Con)
Governing Vessel (Gov)

Twelve Principal Channels
Stomach Channel (Sto)
Spleen Channel (Spl)
Small Intestine Channel (SmI)
Heart Channel (Hea)
Bladder Channel (Bla)
Kidney Channel (Kid)
Pericardium Channel (Per)
Triple Warmer Channel (TrW)
Gall Bladder Channel (GaB)
Liver Channel (Liv)
Lung Channel (Lun)
Large Intestine Channel (LaI)

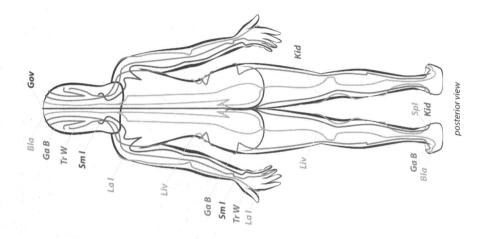

posterior view

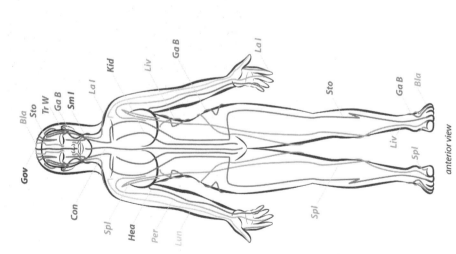

anterior view

Illustration courtesy of Shutterstock.

described, meaning that the channels were duplicated on each side of the body in a mirror image. These paired channels are named for organs of the body. The channels are kidney, heart, small intestine, urinary bladder, spleen, lung, large intestine, stomach, liver, *san jiao*,[15] pericardium,[16] and gallbladder.

The channels can directly influence the named organ, but they also affect other areas and physiological processes. Additionally, eight "extraordinary" channels were noted. These special channels run in various directions, over and through the body, connecting the principal channels and acting as reservoirs of qi. Acupuncture theory is discussed in more detail later in this chapter.

As in all ancient civilizations, the Chinese used indigenous plants, minerals, and animals as medicine. Chinese herbology predates acupuncture, probably by thousands of years, but until the development of written language, the use of these medicinals was not documented. Several very famous texts categorize Chinese herbs and explain their functions. *Shen Nong Ben Cao Jing* (*The Divine Farmer's Materia Medica*) was written in the early Tang dynasty (452–536 CE), but it is actually a compilation of much earlier writings. The book discusses the attributes of 365 herbs, the majority of which are still used today.

Dr. Zhang Zhong Jin (150–219 CE) was renowned for his text, the *Shang Han Lun* (*Treatise on Cold Damage*), the oldest formulary to group patient symptoms into clinically useful categories. Zhang Zhong Jin was also the first to link diagnoses derived through the principles of yin-yang theory and the Wu Xing (Five Phases) with standardized herbal treatments.

One of the most celebrated physicians in the history of Chinese medicine was Dr. Li Shi Zhen, who lived during the Ming dynasty and, in 1578, wrote his masterpiece, the *Ben Cao Gang Mu* (*Compendium of Materia Medica*). Li Shi Zhen traveled across China in search of medicinal herbs. After twenty-seven years of diligent work, the *Ben Cao Gang Mu*

---

15. Also known as Triple Heater or Triple Burner.
16. Also known as Master of the Heart.

was completed. It documents 1,892 distinct herbs and more than eleven thousand formulas. This comprehensive text remained the official materia medica for China for the next four hundred years.

Two other noteworthy Chinese doctors are Hua Tuo (145–203 CE) and Sun Si-Miao (581–683 CE). Hua Tuo was well known, especially for his surgical skills and the development of a particular type of exercises that he called Five Animal Play (Wu Qin Xi). Sun Si-Miao stood out not only for his talent as a healer, but also for his humanity. Although the emperors of the Tang dynasty wanted Sun Si-Miao as the palace physician, he declined and worked for all people. In his writings, he instructed doctors to be of good moral character and to treat all patients equally, regardless of their class or wealth.

Around the time of Sun Si-Miao, during the fifth and sixth centuries, Eastern medicine spread from China to Japan, Korea, and Vietnam. Through trade via the Silk Road, knowledge of this system of medicine eventually arrived in the Middle East and Europe, with little more than passing interest outside Asia until much later. As European colonization of East Asia increased, more Western physicians became curious about these techniques. France had colonized Vietnam, and so French physicians who traveled there were exposed to the successes of acupuncture and herbal formulas. From the eighteenth century onward, the French were at the forefront of Western investigations of Eastern medicine. Later in this chapter, we discuss the science of acupuncture and other Eastern healing modalities in greater detail.

An increasing percentage of the general population has benefited from Eastern medicine over the past century, but in the United States very few were able to take advantage of this powerful medical system prior to the 1970s. Until then, acupuncture was illegal in America. Even though it was utilized and well respected throughout Europe, Britain, Canada, Japan, and other Asian countries, both practitioners and patients who sought to use this medicine risked arrest in the United States. For this reason, very little documentation remains of the early history of Eastern medicine in America. There are, however, some accounts dating as far back as the nineteenth century. In 1974, California became the first state to legalize the practice of acupuncture, after which most other states began to follow suit. Acupuncture training and credentialing became more formalized, but there are still a few states in which there is no acupuncture practice act to regulate the profession. In all states except Hawai'i, a medical doctor or osteopath may practice acupuncture, for which most states require approximately three hundred hours of acupuncture training; such a practitioner is called a medical acupuncturist. A licensed acupuncturist is not usually a medical doctor or osteopath, although some physicians choose to enroll in schools of acupuncture and Eastern medicine. Licensed acupuncturists usually have some postsecondary education and then will have completed approximately three thousand hours of training in acupuncture and herbology. This also would include hundreds of hours of Western biomedicine such as anatomy, biology, chemistry, physiology, and pharmacology.

Whether a medical or licensed acupuncturist, the mark of an excellent practitioner is their willingness to refine the art and science of Eastern medicine. Collaboration among acupuncturists and other health-care practitioners is happening more frequently in clinics, hospitals, and academic institutions. The drive to comprehend the mechanism of action of acupuncture, qigong, tai chi, yoga, and meditation has fueled thousands of basic research studies and clinical trials. In the discussion that follows, we provide a brief summary of the current understanding of how these therapies can heal the human body.

The Science Behind Eastern Healing Modalities

From Asia to Europe to the rest of the world, interest in and use of Eastern medicine has grown during the past century, surging over the last fifty years. Several components of Eastern medicine have been subject to scientific scrutiny in the West, but also in their countries of origin. The elements of Eastern medicine (including Indian, Tibetan, and Chinese practices) that have been most researched are meditation and breath control, yoga, qigong, tai chi, herbal remedies, and acupuncture.

Regulation of the breath has been used for millennia to calm the mind and heal the body. Even without a modern understanding of how the brain and body communicate, the ancients formulated breathing techniques that balanced the autonomic nervous system. This is the part of your brain, nerves, and immune and endocrine systems that determine your state of relaxation. The autonomic nervous system is composed of the sympathetic nervous system and the parasympathetic nervous system. The sympathetic nervous system initiates the release of stress hormones when your brain perceives that you are in danger. These hormones cause your heart rate to elevate, your blood pressure to rise, and makes glucose available to fuel your muscles in preparation for combat or evasive maneuvers. This reaction is known as the fight-or-flight response. In contrast, the parasympathetic nervous system calms all these processes and returns the body to a normal state of activity. Slow, deep breathing stimulates the main nerve of the parasympathetic nervous system, called the vagus nerve, which in turn releases hormones and neurotransmitters that slow your heart rate, lower your blood pressure, and generally bring your body into balance.[17] The benefits of calming the nervous system include decreasing chronic inflammation, thereby decreasing your risk of chronic illness.

Controlling the breath is often one of the first steps employed in meditation. There are many different types of meditation—Buddhist, Hindu, Zen, Tibetan, Daoist, mindfulness, and many more. Depending on the ideology associated with the practice, the goals of meditation can range from relaxation and stress relief to compassion and spiritual enlightenment. Meditation usually results in a sense of calmness and clarity that can be difficult to describe. Numerous medical benefits have

17. T. M. Srinivasan, "Pranayama and Brain Correlates," *Ancient Science of Life* 11 (1/2): 1–6; D. Krshnakumar, M. R. Hamblin, and S. Lakshmanan, "Meditation and Yoga Can Modulate Brain Mechanisms That Affect Behaviour and Anxiety," *Ancient Science of Life* 2 (1): 13–19, doi:10.14259/as/v2i2il1.171; Michael M. Zanoni, "Healing Resonance Qi Gong and Hamanaleo Meditation," https://www.mikezanoni.com /meditation-qi-gong, accessed February 4, 2018.

been attributed to meditation, and scientists are investigating how meditation affects the brain and overall health.

When a person meditates, the electrical activity in the brain changes. This is true of any change of state such as intense concentration or emotion, drowsiness, sleep, and dreaming. These patterns of electrical activity are called brain waves and are measured by electroencephalography (EEG). Brain waves, also known as neural oscillations, have different frequencies. In addition, a wide range of patterns, combinations of frequencies, and amplitudes are associated with different stages of sleep and wakefulness. For instance, you can be awake and in a state of deep concentration as you are trying to solve a problem or you can be awake but daydreaming and inattentive. Each of these states of wakefulness has different patterns involving each of the frequencies, but in different proportions, and can involve different areas of the brain. Simply stated, higher-frequency brain waves are associated with cognitive processing and alertness (beta waves); lower frequencies are associated with sleep (delta waves). In between, there are frequencies associated with wakefulness (alpha waves) and deep relaxation, daydreaming, and meditation (theta waves). Combinations of delta and theta waves are important in memory processing. The state of mind between alpha and theta waves is said to be one of increased creativity.

Through the use of functional magnetic resonance imaging (fMRI), researchers have discovered that meditation increases the amount of gray matter in the brain, which is made up predominantly of the cell bodies of the neurons,[18] and also seems to slow the natural loss of gray matter that occurs as we age.[19] Depending on the location of the gray matter within the brain, it is involved with a variety of functions such as learning, memory, emotional regulation, and per-

18. Britta K. Holzel et al., "Mindfulness Practice Leads to Increases in Regional Brain Gray Matter Density," *Psychiatry Research* 191 (1): 36–43, doi:10:1016/j. pscychresns.2010.08.006.

19. N. Last, E. Tufts, and L. E. Auger, "The Effects of Meditation on Grey Matter Atrophy and Neurodegeneration: A Systematic Review," *Journal of Alzheimer's Disease* 56 (1): 275–286, doi:10.3233/JAD-160899.

spective. It seems that meditation can actually keep your brain younger and calmer.

A meditative state can be achieved during qigong, tai chi, and yoga. All these practices incorporate slow deep-breathing patterns, which confer all the benefits of seated meditation. These forms of moving meditation have additional advantages. During these practices, we move in well-defined patterns, stretching all the muscles in the neck, torso, arms, and legs. Stretching has many benefits, such as decreasing pain, improving blood circulation, increasing range of motion, and improving balance. For some time now, the cellular changes that occur with stretching have been studied. Dr. Helene Langevin and her team at Harvard have demonstrated that by gently stretching the connective tissue of mice, inflammation at a site of injury was reduced. There was also an increase in the concentration of resolvins, the cellular mediators that help coordinate the resolution of the acute inflammatory episode.[20] Later, using a similar rodent model and injecting breast cancer cells into the mice, Dr. Langevin found that gentle connective tissue stretching enhanced the response of the immune system and slowed the tumor growth by half.[21] This finding may offer an explanation for why many researchers have noted a lower risk of death from all causes, including recurrence, in cancer patients who exercise.[22]

An additional benefit of slow-moving, breath-focused exercise relates to the way the body utilizes oxygen. Dr. Peter Anthony Gryffin has compared the amount of oxygen in the blood during and after aerobic exercises such as running and after slow, mindful exercises like tai chi and qigong. It was previously known that the amount of oxygen in the blood, a measurement called blood oxygen saturation, either stays the same or goes down during aerobic exercise as oxygen is being utilized

---

20. L. Berrueta et al., "Stretching Impacts Inflammation Resolution in Connective Tissue," *Journal of Cellular Physiology* 231 (7): 1621–1627, doi:10.1002/jcp.25623.

21. L. Berrueta et al., "Stretching Reduces Tumor Growth in a Mouse Breast Cancer Model," *Scientific Reports* 8:7864, doi:10.1038/s41598-018-26198-7.

22. David O. Garcia and Cynthia A. Thomson, "Physical Activity and Cancer Survivorship," *Nutrition in Clinical Practice* 29 (6): 768–779, doi:10.1177/0884533614551969.

by the large muscle groups, heart, and lungs. During slow-moving, breath-focused exercises, blood oxygen saturation initially goes up, then drops significantly for a short period of time before returning to baseline. Dr. Gryffin's research suggests that this drop in blood oxygen saturation represents increased oxygen metabolism and diffusion throughout the whole body, since no excessive strain is placed on the muscles and cardiovascular system, as occurs during aerobic exercise. Because of this unique difference in oxygen metabolism, Dr. Gryffin coined the term "metarobics" to describe exercises that are neither aerobic, like running or swimming, nor anaerobic, like weight lifting. Metarobic exercises include tai chi, qigong, yoga, and other forms of moving meditation. This improved oxygen metabolism may account for many of the health benefits realized by practitioners of tai chi and qigong, such as decreased levels of chronic inflammation, improved immunity, and enhanced healing.[23]

Along with meditation, breath regulation, and movement, herbs are a mainstay in Eastern medicine, as well as in every medical tradition around the world. The healing properties of plants have been known for thousands of years, but not until the last two hundred years have specific biologically active compounds been extracted and used as drugs. As technology advanced, the medicinal properties of herbs were documented, particularly in China, where sophisticated combinations of herbs are used alongside modern pharmaceuticals in clinics and hospitals that integrate Western and Eastern care modalities. The constituent components of these herbs, the ways they are metabolized, and how they affect the body continue to be documented. These plants have naturally occurring compounds that, depending on the herb, can act as antibacterials, antivirals, antifungals, hormone modulators, neurotransmitters, anti-inflammatories, antidepressants, or sleep aids. It is not within the scope of this book to discuss the biochemistry of all the herbs available to a qualified practitioner, but it should be noted that many of

---

23. Peter Anthony Gryffin, *Mindful Exercise: Metarobics, Healing, and the Power of Tai Chi* (Wolfeboro, NH: YMAA Publication Center, 2018), 15.

the formulas around today have been prescribed effectively in Asia for more than a thousand years.

The concept of using plants as medicines was well established throughout the world, but it was the mystery of acupuncture that fascinated the French. This led to various scientific experiments that laid the foundation for modern acupuncture research.

During the mid-twentieth century, the French and the Chinese performed a number of experiments that began to explain how acupuncture works. There is no single, simple explanation for acupuncture's mechanism of action. Each scientist added new information, helping to fill in the pieces of the puzzle.

In the 1940s and 1950s, Dr. J. E. H. Niboyet designed a series of experiments that showed electrical resistance is lower at acupuncture points than elsewhere on the body. This means electricity will pass into the body more easily across the skin at an acupuncture point than across the skin at a non-acupuncture point. Niboyet also demonstrated that electricity flowed more easily along the same acupuncture channel than between channels that were not as strongly related to each other. These results were confirmed by other scientists in the 1960s and 1970s.[24]

The acupuncture channel itself has remained an elusive entity. Our understanding of acupuncture channels and how acupuncture works has changed over time. Acupuncture channels are intimately associated with the neural, immune, and endocrine systems of the body. For example, modern acupuncture researchers note the channels that run on the inner arms almost exactly follow the paths of the nerves. Though the ancient Chinese were aware of the existence of the structures we call nerves, they did not know their function. They could not have known that electrical signals travel along nerves, having no knowledge of electricity.

Understanding that the effect of acupuncture is mediated via electricity was the first step in uncovering its mechanism of action. Over the past half century, the unfolding of this knowledge began by seeking

---

24. Joseph Helms, *Acupuncture Energetics: A Clinical Approach for Physicians* (Berkeley, CA: Medical Acupuncture Publishers, 1995), 21.

evidence that these channels do exist: they were thought to be different than the known vascular or neurological systems that have been defined by modern medicine. The first piece of indirect evidence of the existence of acupuncture channels is that many patients experience a feeling of heaviness, achiness, or warmth around the acupuncture needles during treatments. These sensations can radiate from the needles, either circumferentially or linearly. When moving linearly, this feeling of warmth or achiness travels up or down the area of the body being needled. Modern Chinese researchers call this phenomenon "propagated sensation along channels."[25] They suggest that this sensation represents the movement of a corrective signal to an area determined by the acupuncture point that has been used. The target zone for the propagated sensation need not be a local area. Needling particular points on an arm or leg can reproducibly create a response in another part of the body. For example, certain points on the hand can alleviate back pain, a point on the lower leg can decrease discomfort of the opposite shoulder, and a well-known combination of points can initiate labor. We do know that the sensations elicited by acupuncture are an essential part of the signaling process and are caused by the activation of different types of nerve fibers.[26]

The speed of the propagated sensation has been noted to travel at one to ten centimeters per second. This velocity varies among subjects and with the intensity of the needling. This rate is much, much slower than the speed of nerve impulses, so it cannot be attributed simply to nerve conduction. The brain itself is also involved in the perception of this sensation. Some studies have reported that amputees who are aware of phantom limbs are able to feel the propagated sensation within the absent limb when needled along a channel associated with the limb in question. This indicates that there must be some central nervous system involvement in the appreciation of this sensation.

---

25. Helms, *Acupuncture Energetics*, 22.

26. Michael Corradino, *Neuropuncture: A Clinical Handbook of Neuroscience Acupuncture*, 2nd ed. (London: Singing Dragon, 2013), 24.

When an acupuncture point is needled, a lot happens on the cellular level. There seems to be another mechanism at play, aside from direct activation of the nervous system. When the needle is inserted, it is manipulated to create sensation. This manipulation causes a mechanical change in the tissue. Researchers have demonstrated, using magnetic resonance imaging and ultrasound elastography, that a slow-moving wave is generated through the tissue that has been needled. There is also a shift in calcium ions that creates a biochemical signal that appears to be separate from the electrical signal of the nerve fibers.[27]

Western science has added a great deal of supporting evidence for the existence of a communication network from acupuncture points to the rest of the body by documenting the effects of acupuncture on blood chemistry, body temperature, and hormone levels. With respect to blood chemistry, acupuncture has been shown to modify levels of glucose, cortisol, triglycerides, and cholesterol. Although the mechanism of action is not well understood, acupuncture seems to assist the body in achieving balance. In medicine, this equilibrium is called homeostasis.

Acupuncture has also been shown to cause an increase in the body's surface temperature, caused by the dilation of vessels, resulting in increased blood flow. The increase has been documented at a rate three times higher than that of pretreatment flow. Not only does the surface temperature of the needled skin increase locally, but it also increases at the same area on the other side of the body.[28] Increased blood flow improves oxygenation within the tissue and may speed healing.

A great deal of research has been performed regarding acupuncture's effect on hormone and neurotransmitter levels, particularly with respect to pain relief. Some of these neurotransmitters include serotonin, norepinephrine, substance P, GABA (gamma-aminobutyric acid), and

27. Edward S. Yang et al., "Ancient Chinese Medicine and Mechanistic Evidence of Acupuncture Physiology," *European Journal of Physiology* 462 (2011): 645–653, doi:10.1007/s00424-011-1017-3.

28. Joseph Helms, *Acupuncture Energetics: A Clinical Approach for Physicians* (Berkeley, CA: Medical Acupuncture Publishers, 1995), 40.

dopamine. All of these compounds work together to diminish the brain's perception of pain.

Another way pain is decreased is through the release of cortisol, which has an anti-inflammatory action. The release of cortisol is controlled by levels of adrenocorticotrophic hormone (ACTH), and acupuncture has been shown to increase the discharge of this substance.

Finally, acupuncture modulates the body's internal production of opioids, leading to pain relief through a different pathway. Opioids are narcotic-like compounds; those produced in the body are called endorphins, which attach to receptors located on cell membranes, resulting in decreased pain. There are several different types of endorphins, and each acts at a different site within the brain and spinal cord to relieve pain. Interestingly, it appears that certain endorphins (beta-endorphin and met-enkephalin) also interact with the immune system. A surge in the levels of these endorphins can lead to increased activity of natural killer cells, a type of white blood cell that defends the body from foreign microbes and cancerous mutations.[29]

For all the various effects that acupuncture produces, the specific mechanism of action has not yet been completely discovered. As we have seen, electricity is a principal mediator of information that is passed along through the body, creating numerous physiologic changes.

Several theories exist regarding the ways in which these processes are regulated. Most of them concentrate on the effects produced by the passage of electrical current through the body. There is no doubt that the human body utilizes electricity in its everyday functioning. Western medicine has used this information to create many diagnostic tests and therapies.

In the heart, the interpretation of the electrical signals seen on an electrocardiogram (EKG) allows a physician to diagnose a heart attack or cardiac rhythm disturbance. If a patient's heart suddenly stops beating, electricity is applied to the person's chest via a device called a defibrillator, in an effort to "kick-start" cardiac activity. Smaller

---

29. Helms, *Acupuncture Energetics*, 41.

amounts of electricity are also used to change irregular rhythms to regular ones.

The electrical signals from the brain can be studied to help diagnose epilepsy or sleep disturbances. We can assess the health of these systems by recording the speed of electrical impulses through the nerves and muscles.

Even skin healing, which we tend to take for granted, requires electricity to activate the restorative process. Electrically, the skin can be described as a battery, with the negative charge inside each cell and the positive charge on the exterior surface. When the skin is breached, either by trauma or by inserting an acupuncture needle, the "battery" is short-circuited, and now the charge on the skin surface is negative. This negative charge seems to be an initiating factor in healing and activates the body's system of repair. It has been shown that this negative charge, described by Dr. Robert Becker as a "current of injury," can last several days following an acupuncture treatment.[30]

Dr. Becker, an American orthopedic surgeon, performed a fascinating series of experiments involving electrical current and limb regeneration in salamanders and frogs. Even though salamanders and frogs are closely related, salamanders can spontaneously regrow lost limbs, but frogs cannot. Through his research, Dr. Becker discovered that the tissue over the salamanders' limb stumps display a relatively negative charge compared with other points on the animal. The frogs did not exhibit this negative charge. When he applied the appropriate electrical current and created a negative charge over the area of the frogs' missing limbs, the frogs' limbs regenerated just like the salamanders' did.[31] Dr. Becker's work has led to the creation of electrical devices that accelerate bone healing. These devices are used in cases in which broken bones are not healing well. In the past, it was sometimes necessary to amputate limbs that would not heal. By using electricity to enhance bone

---

30. Helms, *Acupuncture Energetics*, 67.

31. Richard Gerber, *Vibrational Medicine: The #1 Handbook of Subtle-Energy Therapies*, 3rd ed. (Rochester, VT: Bear and Company, 2001), 91.

healing, Dr. Becker's discovery has decreased the need for amputation in such circumstances.

As well as the electrical component of the energy within the human body, there is also a magnetic constituent. Without this, magnetic resonance imaging (MRI) would not be possible. Studies called functional MRIs are used to observe the electromagnetic changes within different areas of the brain in response to acupuncture needling.

Other devices have been developed that can measure electromagnetic fields that come from diverse parts of the body. Such devices have demonstrated that electromagnetic fields exist around acupuncture points and that the intensity of these fields changes following acupuncture treatment.[32] Some researchers suggest that acupuncture points act as amplifiers by increasing the signal that moves along the channel.

Identifying the exact tissues through which these electromagnetic signals pass is a subject of ongoing study. Evidence suggests a variety of mechanisms through which bioelectrical information is transmitted. These mechanisms include

- Electron-rich fluid that naturally bathes the tissues of the body, organized into tiny pockets now recognized as the interstitium, a newly defined organ[33]
- Perineural cells (cells that are adjacent to nerves)
- Proteins such as hormones and neurotransmitters that regulate communication between cells
- The fascia, a fibrous tissue that surrounds and connects every component of the body, from nerves, arteries, and veins to each muscle and organ

---

32. Joseph Helms, *Acupuncture Energetics: A Clinical Approach for Physicians* (Berkeley, CA: Medical Acupuncture Publishers, 1995), 62.

33. Petros C. Benias et al., "Structure and Distribution of an Unrecognized Interstitium in Human Tissues," *Scientific Reports* 8, article no. 4947, doi:10.1038/s41598-018-23062-6.

In his superb book *The Spark in the Machine,* Dr. Daniel Keown explains the role that fascia plays in the body, including its electrical properties. Fascia is composed of collagen. Collagen is a protein that accounts for 30 percent of the proteins in our body. Proteins are made of amino acids. In collagen fibers, these amino acids are arranged into three threads that twist around each other like three-stranded rope, lending incredible tensile strength to the tissues in which it is found; these include bones, ligaments, tendons, cartilage, arteries, and connective tissue. Just as it sounds, connective tissue connects and surrounds all our organs and muscles. Collagen even creates the lattice of the interstitium and interacts directly with the fluid inside these bundles, potentially allowing communication between body systems.[34]

Dr. Keown explains that, because of its molecular structure, collagen can act like a crystal and generate small currents of piezoelectricity when it undergoes mechanical stress. If a substance is piezoelectric, it will generate a change in electrical charge when it is compressed and then returns to its original shape. We take advantage of piezoelectricity when we use pilot lights on a gas grill to create a spark, igniting the flame. Collagen is also a semiconductor. This means that collagen can conduct electricity, but not as well as metal such as copper. It can also act as an insulator, but not as well as glass. So, with every movement you make, your tendons, muscles, and bones undergo mechanical strain, and the collagen generates an electrical current. Collagen is an integral part of the fascia that connects the top of your head to the tip of your toes. Dr. Keown describes this as "an interconnected, living electrical web."[35]

When an acupuncture needle is inserted into the body, it makes contact with this "living electrical web." The acupuncturist will usually manipulate the needle until both the patient and the practitioner are aware of a certain sensation. The patient may feel an ache or a slight electrical zing at the insertion site, and this feeling may propagate along the body part that is needled. The acupuncturist can feel this through the

34. Benias et al., "Structure and Distribution of an Unrecognized Interstitium."
35. Daniel Keown, *The Spark in the Machine* (London: Singing Dragon, 2014), 21.

needle. This sensation is called "de qi," or "the arrival of the qi." Even if the needle is inserted into an area that is not classified as an acupuncture point or is not along the channel, this sensation may be felt. This is because the fascia wraps the whole body, not only along acupuncture channels. Just as the blood flows through large vessels and tiny capillaries, so too, does piezoelectricity traverse the whole body.

Knowing about the "body electric," researchers have tried to explain the location of acupuncture channels and points, forming hypotheses regarding the way in which bioelectromagnetic information travels through the body. Chang-Lin Zhang and Fritz-Albert Popp theorize that electromagnetic energy travels in waves.[36] These waves bounce off the physical structures in the body such as bones, nerves, and skin, creating interference patterns, similar to the way waves of water reflect off the sides of a pool. As they change direction, the waves combine with others, creating higher waves, or canceling each other out. Zhang and Popp suggest that acupuncture points and channels occur at areas where bioelectromagnetic waves have combined to form new waves of higher amplitudes, and that acupuncture needles can be used to change the body's electromagnetic field.

Acupuncture needles may influence the state of the body through more than one single path. The human body is a complex system, and it seems likely that the ways in which acupuncture affects it are manifold. In an effort to tease apart the specific mechanism of action, researchers over the years have designed studies comparing true acupuncture with different sorts of pretend acupuncture, called sham acupuncture.

Sham acupuncture has been variously described as needling prescribed points superficially, needling non-acupuncture points, needling points that have not traditionally been used for the condition being treated, or using retractable needles to simulate the experience of true acupuncture without the actual needle insertion.

In numerous studies, sham acupuncture has been shown to be almost as effective as true acupuncture. Those that doubt the usefulness

---

36. Helms, *Acupuncture Energetics*, 69.

of acupuncture interpret this as placebo effect; however, when using shallow needling, alternate points, or retractable needles, the collagen in the connective tissue of the body is still compressed. The piezoelectric property of collagen is activated whenever these tissues are compressed, and microcurrents of electricity are generated. The body's response to the energetic input of sham acupuncture may not be as pronounced as when the points are actually needled, but the body responds nonetheless. This explains why, in some studies, sham acupuncture can be better than no treatment and almost as effective as "real" acupuncture, particularly if the sham acupuncture involves skin penetration. One interesting finding in a recent systematic review of acupuncture trials in the treatment of several types of chronic pain is that penetrating sham acupuncture more closely approximates the pain-relieving effect of true acupuncture than does the non-penetrating sham.[37]

Prior to our clearer understanding of the physiological effects of acupuncture, many considered the improvements patients experienced to be the result of a placebo effect, which has been seen in medical practice for centuries. The word "placebo" comes from the Latin meaning "to please." The idea was that a doctor would give a patient a pill or treatment that was inert. If a pill, there was no active substance in it; if a treatment or surgery, there was no actual intentional repair of any structure. In spite of this, a large number of patients actually improved or were cured. Historically, placebos were used to encourage the patient's expectation that they would recover. From a research standpoint, placebos are used in an effort to ensure that the experience that both the study group and control group undergo is as close to the same as possible. This is done in an effort to isolate the one active substance or intervention that is creating a change in the patient's condition. Introducing a placebo group into a randomized controlled trial is a common

37. A. J. Vickers et al., "Acupuncture for Chronic Pain: Update of an Individual Patient Data Meta-Analysis," *Journal of Pain* 19 (5): 455–474, doi:10.1016/j.jpain.2017.11.005.

occurrence, but as we have seen, sometimes placebos confuse rather than clarify the results.

Even when a study involves a simple cause-and-effect response, such as testing a new drug, it is impossible to separate the human reactions of the participants, both patients and researchers. Medical anthropologists, such as Cecil Helman, have pointed out for some time that there is a "total effect" of a drug or intervention that goes beyond the actual biochemical or physiologic nature of the treatment. The components that make up the total effect include the characteristics of the drug or treatment itself (even down to the color of the pill), the characteristics of the patient (age, gender, genetics, education, experience, personality, expectations), the characteristics of the researcher (personality, age, gender, attitude, professional status), and the setting in which the study is taking place.[38]

None of the above attributes can be removed from the clinical trial, and all of these characteristics are present within the study and placebo groups. This may, in part, explain why some patients who receive the active substance experience a negative clinical response and some within the placebo group improve.

So, does this mean that the positive clinical results experienced by placebo group patients are a figment of their imagination? No. In many studies, the improvements seen in the placebo group can be objectively identified. These changes are not just qualitative, meaning the patient describes a state of improved health. The differences can also be defined quantitatively, such as findings of lower blood pressure and lower cholesterol levels, and the decreased use of painkillers.

How can these changes be occurring? There is a great deal of interest in physiologic effects of the placebo. Around the world, researchers are documenting changes that occur in the immune system, the brain, the spinal cord, and the biochemical balance of the body in response to a placebo.

---

38. Elisabeth Hsu, "Treatment Evaluation: An Anthropologist's Approach," in *Integrating East Asian Medicine into Contemporary Health Care*, ed. Volker Scheid and Hugh MacPherson (Edinburgh: Churchill Livingston/Elsevier, 2012), 158.

In many of these studies, patients are not told they are receiving a placebo. For many, this presents an ethical dilemma in the use of placebos in general practice. Interestingly, at Harvard's Program for Placebo Studies, Kaptchuk and others created a randomized controlled trial to look at the feasibility of using placebos without deceiving the patient.[39] All the patients had irritable bowel syndrome (IBS). The patients were randomized either to the open-label placebo group or the nontreatment control. Both groups received the same amount of time, counseling, and attention. Both groups were asked not to change any aspect of their usual routines for the duration of the study, such as starting a new diet or exercise program. Both groups had stable disease. The difference came at the end of the first interview, when the patients found out to which group they were assigned. The open-label group was told the pills they would take were "placebos, made of an inert substance, like sugar pills, that have been shown in clinical studies to produce significant improvement in IBS symptoms through mind-body self-healing processes."

The truly fascinating outcome of Kaptchuk's study was that, even though patients knew they were taking placebos, their IBS symptoms improved more than those of the control group, which did not receive any pills. The statistically significant changes in the study group were decreased symptom severity and increased symptom relief. There was also a trend toward improved quality-of-life scores at the end of the study period for those taking placebos. Remember that these patients knew there was no medication of any sort in their pills, and yet they felt better. This demonstrates that the power of the mind to heal the body is astonishing. Eastern medicine has always recognized that fact and uses it to full advantage by incorporating meditation, qigong, and tai chi into patient care. Further research will shed more light on this intriguing phenomenon. Even though the mechanism of action is not

---

39. T. J. Kaptchuk et al., "Placebos without Deception: A Randomized Controlled Trial in Irritable Bowel Syndrome," *PLoS One* 5 (12): e15591, doi:10.1371/journal.pone.0015591.

fully understood, we can still benefit from the positive physiologic changes that acupuncture and mind-body interventions produce.

Western Health-Care Providers and Eastern Medicine

Conventionally trained physicians all over the world are seeking ways to help their patients move toward optimal health. There is a strong sense among Western health-care providers that pharmaceutical and surgical interventions may not be enough to correct the course of modern diseases, the majority of which are caused by poor lifestyle choices. There is no doubt that under certain circumstances, medications and surgery can be lifesaving; however, medicine often does not get to the root of the problem and only acts as a temporary fix. Increasingly, doctors, physician assistants, and nurse practitioners recommend integrating complementary therapies into regular medical care.

Even without the input of a health-care provider, people are choosing to use supplements, herbs, and treatments that are not considered standard in Western medicine. The National Institutes of Health (NIH) regularly conducts surveys of tens of thousands of adults regarding their use of complementary or alternative medicine; approximately one-third of those surveyed use these therapies. Western practitioners now commonly ask their patients if they are using any other supplements, herbs, or alternative healing modalities. In fact, medical students are now taught to ask these questions as a matter of course, and academic health centers for integrative medicine can be found in such prestigious schools as Harvard, Tufts, Stanford, the University of Toronto, and the Mayo Clinic, to name but a few. Medical students are now learning about other traditional health systems so they can understand how these treatments can be safely integrated into conventional care. Hospitals are also offering complementary and integrative healing services. The American Hospital Association released a survey in 2011 demonstrating that 42 percent of their member hospitals provided these modalities, representing an increase from 37 percent in 2007.[40]

These complementary therapies cover a wide range of options and healing systems. Depending on practitioners' interests and experience, they may suggest adjunctive Western therapies such as biofeedback, relaxation techniques, massage therapy, health coaching, and lifestyle medicine programs. Or they might consider Ayurvedic medicine that incorporates yoga, meditation, herbs, and dietary therapies based on the patient's underlying constitution. Yet again, they may refer their patients to a practitioner of Eastern medicine. Like other healing systems, Eastern medicine is composed of various strands: dietary therapy, exercise, qigong, tai chi, meditation, bodywork, herbal formulas, and acupuncture. All of these complementary therapies are aimed at improving the physical, mental, and emotional health of the patient and modifying underlying behaviors that contribute to chronic disease.

Many medical practitioners and patients will have preferences regarding which therapeutic interventions to use. After discussing the options, they may decide to stick with one traditional system entirely or mix and match depending on circumstances. For example, someone may respond well to Ayurvedic dietary therapy but have mobility problems and find it too difficult to get down on the floor to practice yoga. That person might do better with tai chi or qigong. Both of these Eastern practices will improve strength and balance as well as provide the preparation for meditation that yoga confers.

We too have our preferences. Our training in both Western and Eastern medicine has shown us that these two systems work extremely well together, and we are not alone. Over the span of two decades, the percentage of Western physicians who had a favorable opinion of Eastern

---

40. American Hospital Association, "More Hospitals Offering Complementary and Alternative Medicine Services," September 7, 2011, https://www.aha.org/press -releases/2011-09-07-more-hospitals-offering-complementary-and-alternative -medicine-services.

medicine increased fourfold. In 1998, only 20 percent of respondents held a positive view of Eastern medicine. When the survey was repeated in 2009, that number had exploded to 80 percent![41]

Even the US military has embraced a component of Eastern medicine. In 2007, the US Air Force asked Dr. Joseph Helms, the founding president of the American Academy of Medical Acupuncture, to develop acupuncture protocols to treat conditions commonly found in combat veterans: post-traumatic stress disorder (PTSD) and pain, both acute and chronic. From 2008 to 2013, the US Department of Defense funded medical acupuncture training for hundreds of military doctors under the guidance of Dr. Helms. When this funding was no longer available, Dr. Helms created the Acus Foundation, a not-for-profit charitable organization, to continue training military health-care providers in medical acupuncture. Acus partnered with Nellis Air Force Base, training all the primary-care physicians so that any patient could receive an acupuncture treatment at any visit upon request or recommendation. In the first year of this pilot program, opioid prescriptions dropped by 45 percent, muscle relaxant prescriptions decreased by 34 percent, and $250,000 was saved thanks to fewer referrals to civilian pain-management specialists.[42]

Although you may not have access to a primary-care provider who is also a skilled acupuncturist, you can rest assured that a great many Western physicians are genuinely interested in incorporating Eastern therapies into conventional medical care. Your doctor may already know a number of reputable practitioners of Eastern medicine and would be happy to refer you. Some patients are reluctant to bring up the topic of incorporating Eastern medicine into their usual treatment plan. They are worried that they will offend their doctors. In this day and age, with

---

41. From the keynote address of the 2011 American Academy of Medical Acupuncture Symposium, given by Emmeline Edwards, MD, director of the Division of Extramural Research at the National Center for Complementary and Integrative Health, a component of the NIH, March 2011.

42. Acus Foundation, https://acusfoundation.org/our-programs/teaching/, accessed June 13, 2018.

all the emerging evidence demonstrating the effectiveness of acupuncture, meditative practices, and lifestyle changes, most physicians are open to adding these strategies to regular care. If your doctor *is* offended, we respectfully suggest you find a new primary care provider.

You will not know how your doctor feels about integrating Eastern and Western medicine until you have the conversation. As we discussed in our first book, *True Wellness*, there may be several reasons that your primary care provider has not spoken to you about these modalities. It may be that your doctor doesn't know whether Eastern medicine would be useful for your particular condition. Or she may not have access to reliable practitioners of Eastern medicine to whom she can send you. Or she may not want to suggest a therapy that might incur additional costs to you if your health insurance doesn't cover these services. These reasons should not prevent you from discussing treatment options with your doctor.

To have a meaningful discussion, you should come to the appointment prepared. You need to do a little homework. Since the inception of the internet, most physicians are very comfortable with patients who have done some online research about their illness and are happy to go through the downloaded information with you. If you are going to present your doctor with such information, it is important that it has come from reputable sources. The World Health Organization report on acupuncture is a good place to start. You could also search the websites of several prominent medical centers that offer Eastern medical services and see what conditions they commonly treat.

You should call your health insurance company to see whether Eastern medical services are a covered benefit and, if so, which providers are in the network. If this option is unavailable to you, you can cover the expense yourself, understanding that within three to five treatments you will know whether they are beneficial. If you live near a school of Eastern medicine, there will be a community clinic where you can receive care for a reduced cost.

Now that you have determined for yourself whether Eastern medicine is a suitable modality for your condition and how to access that care, you will feel more comfortable broaching the subject with your doctor. Generally, the situations in which patients explore options outside of biomedicine are those in which the patient is not improving. In cases where the problem is acute, Western treatment options usually solve things quickly. For patients with chronic conditions, healing may be slower and require greater effort on the part of the patient and the physician. Often both parties become frustrated with what appears to be a lack of progress. Eastern medicine is well suited to treating people in such circumstances. As we have mentioned previously, some patients do worry that their doctor would be offended at the suggestion of a complementary therapy, but in truth, that rarely happens. In our experience, most Western practitioners are interested only in their patients' well-being and are delighted at the prospect of successful treatment through Eastern medicine.

Occasionally, in difficult cases where a patient has not improved with conventional treatments, a physician may feel a sense of failure or embarrassment that she has not been able to help that person sufficiently. Following an honest and respectful discussion of Western and Eastern treatment options, often doctors and patients alike are relieved that a new plan has been formulated. Although the Western physician may not be administering the Eastern treatment herself, she would still be a part of your health-care team and would certainly do her best to facilitate this new aspect of your care where possible.

Finally, it is very important that you keep your doctor aware of any non-allopathic treatments that you are undergoing. Even if you have decided on your own to seek the help of an Eastern medical practitioner, your Western doctor needs to know this, particularly if you are taking any herbs or supplements. Many medications can interact with herbs, supplements, and foods, leading to dangerous situations in which the action of the drug is either accentuated or diminished, resulting in medical complications.

Keep in mind that acupuncture and herbs, while extraordinarily effective, are not the only components of Eastern medicine. Acupuncture and herbs are treatments that are given to you by a skilled professional.

But healthy food, moderate exercise, and a quiet mind are the foundation of Eastern medicine, as well as many other healing traditions. Although both your Western and Eastern health-care providers can offer you encouragement and effective strategies for improving your physical and emotional well-being and sleep, only you can enact these changes to achieve optimal health.

CHAPTER 2

The Heart and Blood Vessels in Health and Disease

The Healthy Heart and Vessels

The human heart is a muscular pump located in your chest that sits between, and is connected to, the right and left lobes of your lungs. The heart contracts in a regular pattern to push blood throughout your body via the arteries and smaller vessels. It generates sufficient force to circulate the blood to all your cells, where the oxygen carried by the red blood cells is used for energy production. Nutrients carried within the fluid portion of the blood are used by the cells of your organs and connective tissue. Waste products of cellular metabolism are moved into the blood and carried to the kidneys and liver, where they are processed and removed from your body.

Heart Anatomy

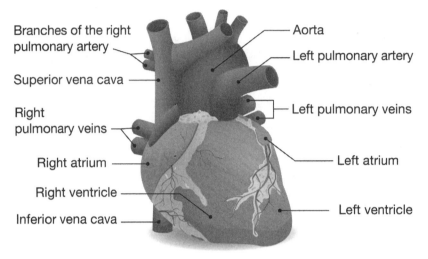

Branches of the right pulmonary artery

Superior vena cava

Right pulmonary veins

Right atrium

Right ventricle

Inferior vena cava

Aorta

Left pulmonary artery

Left pulmonary veins

Left atrium

Left ventricle

Illustration courtesy of Shutterstock.

The pressure generated with each heartbeat is transmitted through all the blood vessels and helps push the blood through the arteries, the organs and connective tissue, and the veins that bring the blood back to the heart. The blood that is carried back to the heart is low in oxygen. It arrives at the first of four chambers of the heart through two large veins called the superior and inferior vena cavae. The superior vena cava carries blood from the upper part of your body and the inferior vena cava carries blood from the lower part. The vena cavae connect to the muscular chamber called the right atrium. When the atrium contracts, it pumps the blood into the right ventricle through a valve that prevents backward flow. Next, the right ventricle contracts, sending blood through another valve into the pulmonary circulation. This circulatory system takes the poorly oxygenated blood to the lungs to pick up oxygen molecules and release carbon dioxide, one of the waste products of your body's metabolism. The freshly oxygenated blood then flows back to the

The Pathway of Blood Flow Through the Heart

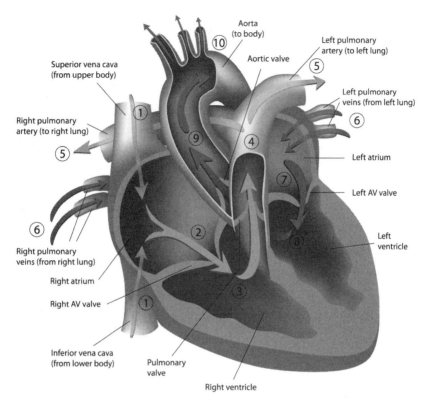

Illustration courtesy of Shutterstock.

heart, this time into the left atrium. From there, it is pumped into the thickly muscled left ventricle. When the left ventricle contracts, it pumps blood into the coronary arteries, to nourish the heart, and into the aorta. The aorta is the largest artery in the body, and it channels blood to smaller and smaller vessels to nourish the entire body.

These four chambers—the right and left atria and the right and left ventricles—contract in a specific sequence to generate movement through the chambers and through the two closed circulatory systems of the lungs and the rest of the body. Each heartbeat actually has two

Human Circulatory System

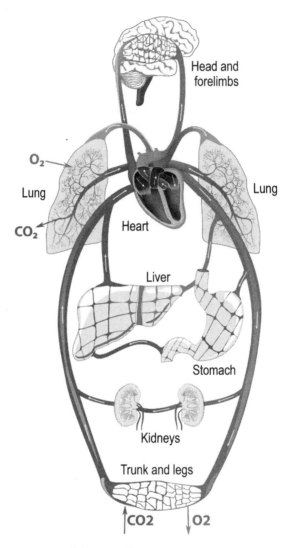

Illustration courtesy of Shutterstock.

components: the right and left atria contract together, and then the right and left ventricles contract together. If you were listening to your heart with a stethoscope, you would hear two sounds. These are the typical "lub, dub" sounds that we all associate with the beating heart. The "lub" portion is the sound of the closing of the valves that separate the atria and the ventricles. The "dub" portion is the sound of the closing of the valves that separate the ventricles and arteries. The pulse you feel when you check your heart rate represents the pressure generated by the left ventricle as it pushes blood into the general (systemic) circulation. There are other heart sounds and variations of heart sounds and pulses that represent different physiological states, but

Work of the Heart Valves

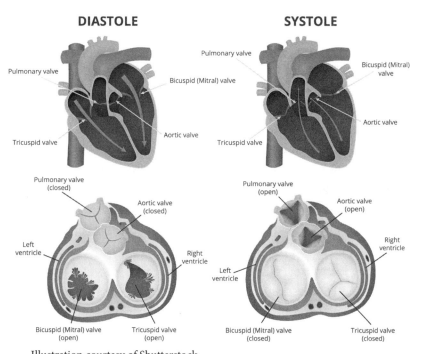

Illustration courtesy of Shutterstock.

knowledge of these entities is not essential for your understanding of the circulatory system.

So, what makes the heart beat? Within the wall of the right atrium is a group of pacemaker cells that form the sinoatrial node. This node is responsible for your heart's natural resting rate. An average resting heart rate is about seventy-two beats per minute. The pacemaker cells produce a spontaneous electrical impulse that travels along the electrical conduction system of your heart and synchronizes the contractions of the muscular heart cells. Remember that each heartbeat has two phases. The cardiac electrical conduction system has a built-in mechanism to ensure that the atria contract before the ventricles do. The electrical signal that causes atrial contractions must go through another node, called the atrioventricular node. Here, the signal is delayed by a tiny fraction of a second to ensure that all the blood is pumped out of the atria and into the ventricles before the ventricles contract. In the event that the sinoatrial node suffers a devastating injury, the atrioventricular node will take over as the heart's pacemaker, though at a much slower rate.

The sinoatrial node fires automatically at your resting heart rate, unless it receives instructions from your brain to speed up or slow down. These messages arrive in the form of neurotransmitters that are released from the two components of your autonomic nervous system, known as the sympathetic and parasympathetic nervous systems. The sympathetic nervous system is responsible for preparing your body to face a perceived threat. When these neurons fire, the neurotransmitters released are norepinephrine (noradrenaline) and epinephrine (adrenaline). This release starts a cascade of preparations; your heart rate increases to supply more blood your body, your lungs relax to take in more air, all the processes involved with digestion are inhibited. In short, your body is preparing to either fight or flee, which is why the activation of the sympathetic nervous system is referred to as the fight-or-flight response. Conversely, activation of the parasympathetic nervous system, which slows your heart rate and promotes digestion, is characterized as the system that allows you to "rest and digest."

Diagram of Electrical System and Nervous System of the Heart

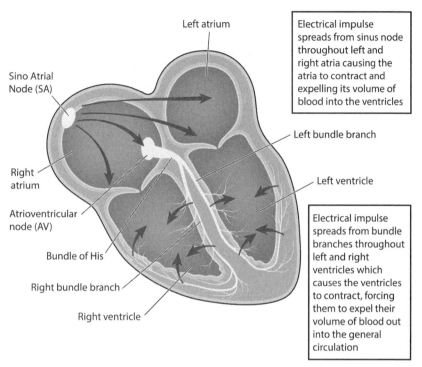

Left atrium

Electrical impulse spreads from sinus node throughout left and right atria causing the atria to contract and expelling its volume of blood into the ventricles

Sino Atrial Node (SA)

Left bundle branch

Right atrium

Left ventricle

Atrioventricular node (AV)

Electrical impulse spreads from bundle branches throughout left and right ventricles which causes the ventricles to contract, forcing them to expel their volume of blood out into the general circulation

Bundle of His

Right bundle branch

Right ventricle

Illustration courtesy of Shutterstock.

The absolute amounts of neurotransmitters received by the heart must be properly balanced. Excessive input from either the sympathetic or parasympathetic neurotransmitters can lead to cardiac injury and even sudden death. Damage to the heart can occur during or after extremely stressful physical and emotional experiences, even in the absence of underlying heart disease. It is indeed possible to die from extreme grief, hopelessness, or overwhelming joy.[1]

Another aspect of your heart rate is garnering increasing attention in cardiac research: the heart rate variability. Heart rate variability refers to the subtle differences in the time between each beat, and it reflects the state of your autonomic nervous system. Previously, your heart rate was considered to be as steady as a metronome, with exactly the same amount of time elapsing from one beat to the next in the resting state. After closer observation, it was noted that the elapsed time actually varies. In the field of obstetrics, this was well known from recording fetal heart rate tracings. By correlating the patterns of fetal heart rate variability with the vigor of newborn babies, it was determined that certain levels of fetal heart rate variability on tracings recorded while the mother was in labor could predict of the well-being of the baby at birth. Though not perfectly predictive, low fetal heart rate variability was correlated with poor vigor and potential neurological damage. If the fetal heart rate variability is too high, there may be cause for concern, but the correlation is not as strong as if the variability is low or absent. In children and adults, there is normally some variability in the heart rate. Research over the past few decades has noted that low heart rate variability indicates a relative predominance of the sympathetic fight-or-flight nervous system and may be associated with increased risk of anxiety, worsening depression, heart disease, and poor outcomes for those with chronic medical conditions.[2]

Communication between the brain and the heart is not just "top down" messaging. Although it has been well documented that neurotransmitters from the brain modulate the function of the heart, the reverse is also true. Specialized sensors called baroreceptors are present in the heart and blood vessels that measure the pressure within these structures. This information is relayed back to the brain, resulting in adjustments of the autonomic nervous system in order to maintain ap-

2. Preeti Chandra et al., "Relationship between Heart Rate Variability and Pulse Wave Velocity and Their Association with Patient Outcomes in Chronic Kidney Disease," *Clinical Nephrology* 81 (1): 9–19; Marcelo Campos, "Heart Rate Variability: A New Way to Track Well-Being," *Harvard Health Publishing*, November 22, 2017, https://www.health.harvard.edu/blog/heart-rate-variability-new-way-track-well-2017112212789.

propriate blood pressure throughout the body. Chemoreceptors in the aorta and carotid arteries measure the amounts of oxygen and carbon dioxide in the blood. These data are also sent to your brain, and changes in respiratory rate, heart rate, and the strength of each cardiac contraction are adjusted, if needed.

Baroreceptor Reflex

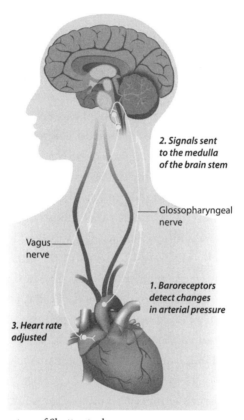

Illustration courtesy of Shutterstock.

The heart is also an endocrine organ, like a gland such as the thyroid, secreting hormones called atrial natriuretic peptide (ANP) and brain natriuretic peptide (BNP) from cells in the atria and ventricles, respectively. Brain natriuretic peptide is actually a misnomer: these peptides are secreted in response to the chambers of the heart being overstretched by too much blood volume. They decrease the volume of the blood by interacting with receptors in the kidneys and causing increased urination and excretion of salts.

In the next section we provide a brief introduction to abnormal conditions of the heart and blood vessels. We then look at each disorder in depth in the following chapters and offer recommendations that integrate Eastern and Western approaches to these conditions.

But First, a Word about Sleep . . .

It may seem odd to interject several pages about sleep in the midst of a book about the heart, but we want to draw your attention to the extreme importance of sleep in the maintenance of cardiovascular health. Many large observational studies have followed millions of patients for decades, and they all report a causal relationship between short sleep and premature death from all causes, including heart disease.[3]

Americans tend to "burn the candle at both ends." Not only is our workweek longer than that of many other industrialized countries, but also our vacations are shorter. Also, Americans tend to stay awake late into the night, usually watching TV or surfing the internet. Not to mention all the people who are required to work night shifts. This schedule has always applied to first-responders like the police, firefighters, hospital staff, and military personnel; however, with the advent of twenty-four-hour shops and services, the number of people who deal with disrupted sleep schedules has ballooned. All this activity takes time away from sleep.

In 2013, the average number of hours we slept in the United States was six and a half hours per night. This is much less than the eight-hours-per-night average documented during the 1950s.[4] According to the CDC, more than 30 percent of Americans get fewer than seven hours of

---

3. Matthew Walker, *Why We Sleep* (Scribner: New York, 2017), 164.
4. Russell Foster, "Why Do We Sleep?" TED Talk, June 2013, http://www.ted.com/talks/russellfosterwhydowesleep.html.

sleep each night.[5] For teenagers, it is even worse. They require nine hours of sleep every night, and many are consistently getting only five!

An hour or so less sleep each night doesn't sound like such a big deal, and it might not be if it were just once in a while. The problem is the cumulative effect of getting too little sleep. Many people do not realize how important sleep is to our neurological, endocrine (hormonal), and immune systems. Lack of sleep has been associated with chronic inflammation,[6] increased cardiovascular disease, decreased immunity, and disrupted hormone secretions, which affect not only our sleep/wake cycle, but also the way our bodies metabolize energy and heal. Chronic sleep disruption has even been designated as a risk factor for cancer. Adequate sleep is critical to brain processing and memory consolidation. During sleep, special channels in certain brain cells open to allow waste products and toxins to drain, thereby keeping the brain functioning well.[7] Inadequate sleep has been associated with the abnormal expression of more than seven hundred genes.[8] This in turn can affect the way the body replenishes itself and, ultimately, lead to degenerative diseases.

The common underlying factor among all these disrupted physiological processes is the imbalance in the autonomic nervous system that is caused by sleep deprivation. As we discussed in chapter 1, the autonomic nervous system is made up of two branches, the sympathetic and the parasympathetic. The sympathetic nervous system is responsible for preparing your body to either fight or flee in order to survive. In contrast, the parasympathetic nervous system calms all the systems in the body and allows it to rest and recuperate. Almost every experiment that

---

5. Centers for Disease Control, "Sleep and Sleep Disorders," https://www.cdc.gov/sleep/data_statistics.html.

6. Janet M. Mullington, Norah S. Simpson, Hans K. Meier-Ewert, and Monida Haack, "Sleep Loss and Inflammation," *Best Practice and Research: Clinical Endocrinology and Metabolism* 24 (5): 775–784, doi:10.1016/j.beem.2010.08.014.

7. Norman Doidge, *The Brain's Way of Healing* (New York: Penguin, 2015), 112.

8. *Huffington Post*, "Sleep Deprivation Affects Genes," February 26, 2013, http://www.huffingtonpost.com/2013/02/26/sleep-deprivation-genesn2766341.html.

has looked at insufficient sleep over the last fifty years has documented an overactive sympathetic nervous system.[9] This means a decrease in the influence of the parasympathetic nervous system, which would normally allow your heart rate and blood pressure to lower during sleep. When your heart and blood vessels are sleep deprived, your heart beats faster and harder and your blood vessel walls constrict, raising your blood pressure and causing strain on the whole system. On top of that, your overactive sympathetic nervous system instructs your adrenal glands to release the stress hormone cortisol, which further narrows your blood vessels.[10] Cortisol also drives the cycle of chronic inflammation that we now know is major factor in all chronic diseases.

If that weren't enough, lack of sleep decreases the levels of growth hormone that your body creates normally during the night. Growth hormone is instrumental in the healing processes of the body. Without sufficient amounts of it, your body will not properly repair the lining of your blood vessels from the usual wear and tear caused by blood coursing through your arteries and veins. Now, if you are sleep deprived, these blood vessels are facing extra strain because of your increased blood pressure and heart rate. It is like a multipronged attack that degrades the insides of all your vessels and makes them more susceptible to plaque formation.[11] Of course, the plaque will be unstable because of the high levels of chronic inflammation brought about by your overactive sympathetic nervous system. Such plaques are more likely to rupture, leading to heart attack and stroke.

In his book, *Why We Sleep*, Dr. Matthew Walker discusses the ultimate sleep experiment. Every March, when those of us in the Northern Hemisphere "spring forward" one hour into daylight savings time, there is a sudden increase in heart attacks, according to the data drawn from millions of hospital records. Conversely, in autumn, when we "fall back"

9. Matthew Walker, *Why We Sleep* (Scribner: New York, 2017), 167.
10. Walker, *Why We Sleep*, 168.
11. Walker, *Why We Sleep*, 168.

one hour, there is a sharp drop in heart attacks.[12] Imagine losing that one hour or more every single night of the year. Imagine the toll it is taking on your body, not just your heart, but also all aspects of every biological system, down to your DNA and genetic expression.

For centuries upon centuries, Eastern medicine has been concerned about sleep quality as it relates to overall health. At last, Western science is starting to catch up. Sleep scientists like Dr. Walker are sounding the alarm about the cost of our societal disregard for sleep because, once chronic sleep deprivation has begun, it is a difficult cycle to break. It is better to recognize inappropriate sleep habits and correct them before it is too late and insomnia sets in. To decrease your risk of heart disease and other chronic conditions caused by insufficient sleep, incorporate the following recommendations into your daily routine:[13]

- Exercise regularly, performing both cardiovascular exercise and "meditative" exercises such as tai chi, qigong, or yoga that will promote relaxation.
- Minimize the use of stimulants (like caffeine) and sedatives (like alcohol or sleeping pills).
- Keep a regular sleep/wake schedule by waking up at about the same time every day, getting exposure to morning light, dimming your lights and avoiding all electronic devices an hour or two before bed, and going to bed at around the same time each night.
- Use your bedroom only for sleep or sexual activity, and banish all electronic devices such as televisions, computers, and cell phones.
- Sleep in complete darkness.
- Pay attention to recurring dreams or nightmares. They may be trying to tell you something important!

---

12. Walker, *Why We Sleep*, 168.

13. Rubin Naiman, "Insomnia," in *Integrative Medicine*, ed. David Rakel, 3rd ed. (Philadelphia: Saunders/Elsevier, 2012), 231.

- If you cannot sleep after lying in bed for fifteen minutes, get up and do something restful, like meditating or taking a warm bath; then try again. Do not lie awake in bed watching the clock!
- Find healthy, constructive ways to manage stress, such as exercise, socializing with family and friends, meditation, qigong, and tai chi.
- Consult your physician if you have persistent difficulty sleeping.

Reducing your risk for chronic, debilitating disease is well within your capability. Even if you are already affected by a chronic condition, you can take control of your lifestyle choices and make a positive impact on your health. Taking steps to balance your autonomic nervous system will reduce the levels of chronic inflammation in your body and support the health of your cardiovascular system. This is a modern way of saying what the ancient Chinese have always advocated; that is, follow the middle road and moderate your habits to improve the flow of blood and qi. Either way you say it, you will be well on the way toward vibrant health and healing.

An Overview of Cardiovascular Disease

The term "cardiovascular disease" or "heart disease" is a general one that describes problems that involve the heart and blood vessels. Heart disease is the most common cause of death in the United States. The Centers for Disease Control and Prevention (CDC) estimates the number of deaths that occur each year and lists the causes, in order of frequency: heart disease consistently holds first place, followed closely by cancer in the number two spot. This is true for both men and women.[14]

Deaths from heart disease alone account for 25 percent of the annual deaths in America, amounting to approximately 600,000 people each year. The costs, both direct and indirect, total $190 billion annu-

---

14. "Deaths, Percent of Total Deaths, and Death Rates for the 15 Leading Causes of Death in 5-Year Age Groups, by Race and Sex: United States, 2010," http://www.cdc .gov/nchs/data/dvs/LCWK1_2010.pdf; "Groups, by Race and Sex: United States, 2010," http://www.cdc.gov/nchs/data/dvs/LCWK1_2010.pdf.

ally. This includes not just the price of treating people with heart disease, but the additional costs associated with loss of productivity.

Heart disease includes

- hardening and narrowing of the arteries (arteriosclerosis/atherosclerosis)
- chest pain (angina)
- heart attack (myocardial infarction, also known as an MI, during which heart muscle dies due to lack of oxygen)
- heart failure (in which the heart can't efficiently pump blood)
- abnormal heartbeat (arrhythmia)
- infections of the heart itself (myocarditis) or heart valves (rheumatic heart disease)
- abnormal vascular structure (e.g., mitral valve prolapse)
- high blood pressure (hypertension)

Each of these conditions can affect the functioning of the circulatory system. Sometimes one condition can lead to the development of another. For example, arteries naturally "harden" with age (arteriosclerosis), but narrowing of the caliber of the vessel is a consequence of cholesterol-filled plaques that stick to the artery wall (atherosclerosis). It is thought that this narrowing is caused by a combination of chronic inflammation and a poor diet, laden with unhealthy fats.

When blood vessels outside of the heart contain plaques, this condition is called peripheral vascular disease (PVD), and atherosclerosis found in the brain is known as cerebral vascular disease (CVD). When atherosclerotic plaques are found in the blood vessels that supply the heart, it is called coronary artery disease (CAD). If these arteries become too narrow, the heart does not receive a sufficient amount of blood, depriving the heart cells of oxygen. This lack of oxygen can result in damage to the heart muscle, which is commonly felt as chest pain (angina pectoris). Angina can also be caused by spasms of the coronary arteries. The arteries may even become entirely blocked by plaque or even by blood clots.

Progression of Artherosclerosis

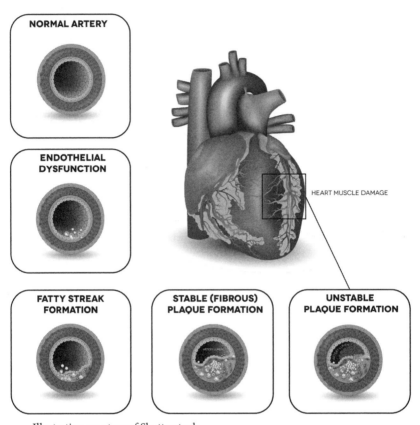

Illustration courtesy of Shutterstock.

Recently, it has been determined that the plaque itself may not be as dangerous as the inflammation. As we discussed in our first book, *True Wellness*, chronic inflammation is at the root of many diseases. When long-term inflammation is present, the plaque is more likely to rupture, sending shards of plaque farther down the vessels that oxygenate the heart. As the body attempts to sequester these bits of plaque, it forms blood clots around them. It is actually the blood clots that can interrupt blood flow to the heart muscle, leading to insufficient oxygenation. If the lack of oxygen is severe enough, heart tissue will start to die (heart attack/MI). Since this tissue is made of muscle, the heart will not be able to pump effectively, and heart failure can occur. Abnormal heart rates can also arise if the damaged area is part of the electrical structure of the heart that controls the rhythm of your heartbeat. As in any complex system, if one component becomes damaged, all other components can be affected.

In chapter 3, we further explain the components of cardiovascular disease and how to best integrate modalities of Eastern and Western medicine to treat these conditions.

The True Wellness Approach to Cardiovascular Disease

I N WORKING AND REWORKING THE ORDER of the sections within this chapter, it occurred to us that the difficulty we were having with the East/West juxtaposition of individual cardiovascular conditions was emblematic of the differences in approach between Western and Eastern medical systems. As discussed in chapter 1, Western medicine has a tendency to reduce a problem to a single cause, with the intent of finding a single solution. Eastern medicine takes a broader view and a whole-systems approach, employing strategies to balance all the organs and functions of the body, encouraging and maximizing our innate ability to heal. Western medicine has gradually been adopting a wider understanding of the multiple, complex causes of heart disease and is becoming more open to the wisdom of Eastern medicine in solving these difficult problems. That is why the True Wellness approach to health combines the best of both systems, using Eastern modalities to prime the body, mind, and spirit to promote overall well-being and utilizing Western discoveries in biochemistry, electrophysiology, and surgery as needed. To help you visualize the integration of Eastern and Western medicine, we have included the "East & West" diagram.

East and West

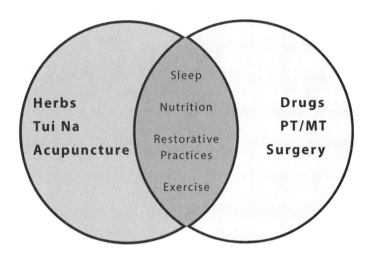

Both health-care systems encourage the optimization of lifestyle behaviors, including sufficient sleep, good nutrition, restorative practices like meditation or qigong, and exercise. The emphasis on these practices has shifted over the millennia. Ancient Western physicians prescribed these components of a healthy lifestyle, but from the time of the Scientific Revolution until recently, such practices were not as actively promoted by conventional health-care providers as they had been in the past. In contrast, Eastern physicians have always taken a whole-systems approach and sought to improve the overall well-being of the patient through these modalities. They understood that the foundational components of good health must be solid in order for the patient to heal. During the past several decades, Western medicine has returned to this perspective. Both paradigms realize that interventions, whether herbs and acupuncture or drugs and surgery, will not be effective in restoring health if a patient's underlying lifestyle foundation is crumbling.

In order to discuss an integrated approach to cardiovascular disease, we have to think in both specifics and generalities. Very often, the best way to solve a specific medical problem is to optimize the general health of the patient, reserving interventions for emergencies or for those patients who need extra assistance to recuperate.

Trying to discuss the Western approach and then the Eastern approach for each condition is cumbersome, owing to the general whole-systems methodology of Eastern medicine. Although Western medicine strives to take that same viewpoint, it is still quite a reductionistic paradigm. So, for clarity, we have divided this chapter into three sections: the Western explanations of various aspects of cardiovascular disease and specific conventional treatments, the Eastern approach to heart health and wellness, and an integrated summary of actionable items for you to use, whether you are recovering from, or trying to prevent, heart disease.

Western Approach to Cardiovascular Disease

Hypertension

Hypertension is another word for high blood pressure within your arteries. Blood pressure assessments actually measure two pressures, measured in millimeters of mercury (mm Hg). One measurement, called the systolic blood pressure, is the highest pressure in the artery at the maximum strength of a heartbeat. The other measurement, called the diastolic blood pressure, is the pressure within the artery when it is at rest *between* heartbeats. Your blood pressure is reported as the systolic blood pressure over the diastolic blood pressure. For example, a normal blood pressure would be 120/80.

Some adults have blood pressures as low as 90/60, and for them, this is normal. A reading of above 140/90 on two separate occasions is considered hypertension; above 180/110 is considered a hypertensive crisis. A gray zone has been categorized as "prehypertension": if your systolic blood pressure is between 121 and 139, or your diastolic blood pressure is between 81 and 89, you have prehypertension.

Why are all these numbers important?

Many people with prehypertension and hypertension have no symptoms at all and feel perfectly well, but having any level of persistently elevated blood pressure increases the risk of heart disease and stroke. Even people with prehypertension have double the risk of developing heart disease than does someone with normal blood pressure. Knowing your blood pressure gives you the opportunity to take action if it is elevated and avoid the complications of hypertension, such as heart attack, stroke, and kidney failure.

High blood pressure is extremely common. According to statistics gathered by the American Heart Association, nearly 80 million adults in the United States have hypertension. That's about one-quarter of the population, and that is not even counting the increasing number of hypertensive children and adolescents! In the decade from 1999 to 2009, the death rate from hypertension increased by 17 percent. The estimated annual cost to the country due to hypertension is more than $50 billion. Clearly, there is a lot of room for improvement.

So, if you have high blood pressure, what can you do? First, you need to understand that some people with hypertension have a genetic predisposition to it. They may be able to make significant improvements in their blood pressure readings through lifestyle changes, but may still require lifelong medication. This should not be considered a failure, at all. Also, the older you are, the more likely you are to have high blood pressure, because your arteries become less pliable. That alone can result in hypertension. Over 65 percent of people sixty-five years old and older have hypertension and, even if your blood pressure is normal at age fifty-five, you still have a 90 percent lifetime risk of becoming hypertensive.

Genetic heritage and aging are factors that you cannot modify, but there are factors that you *can* change. If you smoke, stop. If you don't exercise regularly, start. If you are overweight, lose ten pounds. Even this relatively small loss can improve your blood pressure significantly. If you eat excessive amounts of salty, highly processed food, change your diet. All these interventions have been shown to significantly decrease blood pressure. Even a small decrease in blood pressure can yield large results. If you lower your systolic blood pressure by 5 mm Hg, for example from 140 to 135, you will lower your chances of dying from the complications of hypertension by 7 percent.

High blood pressure can also be caused by stress, being overweight, drinking too much alcohol, and insulin resistance. Certain medications can increase blood pressure, such as birth control pills and some decongestants. Particular herbs can also cause hypertension. These include ephedra, panax ginseng, and excessive amounts of licorice. Your healthcare provider should be asking you about all your medications, supplements, and herbal remedies, in order to determine whether these have any bearing on your hypertension.

Read through the following segments regarding the Western and Eastern management of hypertension. If your only chronic condition is high blood pressure, look at it as an early warning sign. If you are able to control your blood pressure with these recommendations, you decrease your risk for even more serious conditions. If you are already taking antihypertensives, you may be able to reduce your medication dosage with your doctor's approval.

Never stop your blood pressure pills without guidance from your doctor, no matter how well you feel. Suddenly stopping such medications could lead to very high blood pressures and, possibly, a stroke.

Because hypertension is so closely linked to heart disease, many of the recommendations are similar. Adequate sleep, stress reduction, smoking cessation, a healthful diet, exercise, and loss of excess weight are key elements in controlling high blood pressure. Supplements, botanicals, and mind-body techniques are also very useful. Of course, antihypertensive medications are crucial for those unable to achieve optimal blood pressures with complementary approaches alone. Let's take a more detailed look at each of these components.

Lifestyle Changes

Sleep

As we have previously discussed, insufficient sleep increases your risk for all chronic diseases, including hypertension, in an inversely correlated fashion. Simply put, the less you sleep, the greater your risk of disease. Make whatever changes are necessary to ensure you sleep restfully for at least seven hours each night. Follow the recommendations we listed in chapter 2 and seek help from your medical provider as needed.

Stress Reduction

In the 1970s, an American cardiologist named Dr. Herbert Benson and his colleagues[1] conducted a number of experiments showing that people could lower their blood pressure by using breathing techniques to induce relaxation and reduce stress. He called this physiological state the "relaxation response." In essence, Dr. Benson was teaching people to meditate but removing any connection to religious or spiritual ideologies. Subsequently, thousands of studies have corroborated the beneficial effects the relaxation response has on hypertension, other cardiovascular conditions, and overall health. We discuss similar methods for reducing stress in the chapters ahead.

Chronic stress has been linked to all sorts of illnesses, not just those related to the heart. It is estimated that between 75 and 90 percent of all doctors' visits for evaluation and treatment are for signs and symptoms related to stress. Whole books have been written about how to reduce your stress levels, and we touch on many of these techniques throughout the following pages. These techniques can help you decrease your blood pressure and your risk for other cardiovascular diseases.

Smoking

For anyone who smokes and has high blood pressure, smoking cessation should be paramount. Smoking increases your risk of complications from hypertension above and beyond the risks of high blood pressure alone. This means an even greater risk of heart attack and stroke. The risk is directly proportional to the amount you smoke: the more you smoke, the higher the risk.

There is no doubt that it is difficult to stop smoking, but help is available in many forms. Most health insurance companies offer smoking cessation programs. There may also be publicly funded programs in your area. It is definitely more cost effective for both the public and private

---

1. Ruanne K. Peters, Herbert Benson, and John M. Peters, "Daily Relaxation Response Breaks in a Working Population II: Effects on Blood Pressure," *American Journal of Public Health* 67 (10): 954–959, PMCID: PMC1653726.

sector to help you quit smoking than to pay for your medical care when you have a heart attack. There are even medications your doctor can prescribe to help you quit. Your health-care provider should be offering you suggestions and encouragement toward this very important goal. Additionally, acupuncture can be used as an adjunctive therapy to help decrease the desire to smoke. It may take you several attempts to finally quit, but it is well worth the effort.

Diet

You may have heard of the DASH diet (Dietary Approaches to Stop Hypertension). This regimen was designed by the National Heart, Lung, and Blood Institute. It was created specifically to control high blood pressure and many, many studies have proven that it does. People with high blood pressure who follow the DASH diet will lower their systolic blood pressure by more than 11 mm Hg and their diastolic blood pressure by more than 5 mm Hg. Moreover, this diet can help you lose weight and decrease levels of low-density lipoproteins (LDL), triglycerides, and fasting blood sugars. All these reductions will further lower your risk for heart disease. As a bonus, the DASH diet can increase the levels of high-density lipoproteins (HDL), a type of cholesterol that can protect against cardiovascular disease.

As with other diets that promote heart health, like the Mediterranean diet and the anti-inflammatory diet, the DASH diet emphasizes vegetables, fruits, and whole grains, and limits saturated fats from animal and dairy sources. The DASH diet may also decrease levels of chronic inflammation in the body, but this is not its primary goal. The main difference between the DASH diet and the Mediterranean or anti-inflammatory diet is that the DASH diet restricts sodium intake to a greater degree than do the other eating plans.

Sodium is directly related to blood pressure. Sodium causes water retention. This is important to the normal cell physiology, but too much sodium results in too much water in your body, which increases the pressure within your blood vessels and causes your heart to work harder. Generally speaking, the more sodium you eat, the higher your blood pressure will be. The higher your blood pressure, the higher your risk for heart attack, stroke, and kidney disease.

We all need some sodium to keep us healthy, but the average American diet contains way too much! The minimum amount of sodium we need to keep our bodies functioning correctly is between 180 and 500 mg each day. It has been estimated that, on average, Americans actually eat roughly 3,500 mg daily. That is seven to twenty times more than we really need! You may be eating this much sodium without even realizing it. Fast foods, restaurant foods, and highly processed foods are all packed with large amounts of sodium.

So if 180 mg/day of sodium is the minimum, and 3,500 mg/day is excessive, how much sodium should you consume each day? Well, that depends on whether you have risk factors for hypertension, already have high blood pressure, or are simply planning to eat sensibly. If you have hypertension, diabetes, or chronic kidney disease, are African American or are over fifty-one years old, you should consume no more than 1,500 mg of sodium/day. If you have none of these risks factors, you may consume as much as 2,300 mg of sodium each day without any adverse result. The American Heart Association has even stricter advice, endorsing only 1,500 mg of sodium/day for all adults.

The DASH diet takes this advice into consideration. The "Standard" DASH diet limits sodium to 2,300 mg daily and the "Lower Sodium" DASH diet advocates 1,500 mg daily. The National Institutes of Health provides a free online guide with a complete list of DASH diet recommendations. You can find the website address in our section of recommended reading and resources.

Adherence to the Mediterranean diet or anti-inflammatory diet can also improve hypertension. These diets have not been studied as extensively as the DASH diet with respect to high blood pressure alone, but all three diets can improve your health in many ways. Each of these eating plans emphasize foods rich in fiber, vitamins, minerals, antioxidants, and unsaturated fats that can decrease chronic inflammation within the body, as well as improve hypertension. It has even been shown that consuming small daily amounts of dark chocolate (at least 70 percent cocoa) and red wine can modestly lower blood pressure.

Still on the subject of food, garlic has also been shown to be helpful in treating hypertension. You can eat one or two cloves of crushed raw garlic daily or use a supplement. Keep in mind that garlic acts as a blood thinner and can interact with medications that have the same purpose, or can affect platelet function.

Whatever dietary modifications you make to lower your blood pressure, the key is to find a style of healthy eating that you will continue for the rest of your life.

Supplements

Several supplements have been researched to determine their ability to lower blood pressure; however, coenzyme Q_{10} (CoQ_{10}) appears to be the only one that has been definitively shown to be helpful. Many studies have looked separately at calcium, magnesium, potassium, and vitamin D supplementation. Population-based studies demonstrate that low levels of these compounds are associated with hypertension and heart disease, but research that has looked at whether supplements of these compounds will lower high blood pressure have yielded inconsistent results. This may have to do with how the studies were designed, whether the people enrolled in the studies were deficient in these minerals or vitamin D in the first place, or even whether the form of the supplement was easily digested or utilized within the cells. It may be that eating foods rich in these substances will lower blood pressure better than taking supplements.

The data on CoQ_{10} is clearer. CoQ_{10}, also known as ubiquinol, is crucial for energy production throughout the body, but particularly in the heart. It is a very effective antioxidant and, as such, reduces oxidative stress that could lead to hypertension and a host of other chronic conditions. Numerous studies have shown that CoQ_{10} supplementation can lower blood pressure, including several randomized controlled trials that demonstrated a reduction in systolic blood pressure of more than 16 mm

Hg and a drop in diastolic blood pressure of greater than 8 mm Hg. Some people in the studies were even able to discontinue blood pressure medications.

If you take CoQ_{10}, do not alter your medication dosage without your doctor's advice. Though the side effects of CoQ_{10} are uncommon, it can be associated with gastrointestinal upset, rash, and headache. CoQ_{10} may also have an anti-platelet effect, so should not be taken with blood thinners unless your doctor has approved. Additionally, patients with liver or gall bladder problems should use caution with CoQ_{10}, as it is processed primarily by the liver and excreted through bile. Your health-care provider can recommend a dose between 75 and 350 mg daily, best taken with a meal that contains some fat.

Herbs

Hawthorn has been used in many cultures around the world for at least two thousand years to treat heart disease and digestive problems. The leaves, flowers, and berries of the hawthorn plant have high levels of flavonoids and flavanols. Concoctions of these various parts not only make your heart beat more strongly but also cause your blood vessels to relax. It is this relaxation that lowers your blood pressure.

Hawthorn is commonly used in Europe and has been incorporated into many Chinese herbal formulas to improve heart function, normalize blood pressure, and alleviate indigestion. Known in China as Shan Zha, the berries of the hawthorn plant are often prepared with sugar and eaten as a sweet snack.

Many different products provide standardized doses of hawthorn. Generally speaking, the dose is between 250 and 500 mg, two to three times a day. As with any supplement or botanical, you should tell your physician if you are planning to use hawthorn.

Exercise

Time and time again, exercise has been shown to be beneficial in treating many chronic illnesses. Hypertension is no exception. Exercise is one of the first-line treatments for high blood pressure. Of course, you will need your doctor's supervision before starting an exercise program. You may need further evaluation of your heart before you begin. Provided that your heart is good shape, you will find exercise extremely helpful in controlling and improving your hypertension.

The American College of Sports Medicine recommends that you exercise moderately for at least thirty minutes on most days of the week, focusing on cardiovascular exercise. You should be able to talk while you are exercising but should be working hard enough that you don't have enough breath to sing. It is also valuable to include two sessions of weight training during the week.

Mind-Body Therapies

The effectiveness of mind-body therapies in decreasing blood pressure lies in their ability to balance the sympathetic and parasympathetic nervous systems, decreasing the fight-or-flight response. Qigong, tai chi, yoga, and meditation have all been shown to decrease high blood pressure. In the randomized controlled trials that have been performed, some patients were even able to stop at least one blood pressure medication.

Heart Attack

Symptoms of a heart attack include the sensation of crushing pressure in the chest or upper abdomen. The pain can be sharp or dull and can sometimes feel like it is traveling up the neck or down the left arm. This can be accompanied by shortness of breath, feeling faint or dizzy, sweating, nausea, and vomiting. It is very important to note that women may not experience typical symptoms during a heart attack. They may feel symptoms that can easily be confused with gastrointestinal problems. A woman may be more likely to dismiss her symptoms as nothing more than an upset stomach. Or, even if she does seek medical attention, a doctor may not immediately think she is having a heart attack. Either way, the diagnosis can be delayed, losing more heart muscle as time goes by. Male or female, it is very important to seek medical attention for any of these symptoms.

Symptoms and Treatment of Heart Attack

First and foremost, if you are having symptoms of a heart attack, seek medical attention immediately. Earlier treatment is associated with better long-term outcomes. No medical provider would scoff at you for seeking treatment for acute symptoms such as chest pain or shortness of breath. Even if it turned out that you had heartburn rather than a heart attack, it is better to be safe than sorry.

If, unfortunately, you are having a myocardial infarction (MI, or heart attack), you will be given medications to normalize your blood pressure and improve the flow of oxygen to your heart. There are medications can that raise your blood pressure and others that can lower it. You would be given whichever drug is necessary. Other medications can relax blood vessels and increase their caliber, allowing oxygen-rich blood to flow through more easily. Another special class of drugs can actually break up clots within your arteries to increase blood flow. Not everyone is a candidate for these clot-busting medications, as they can have severe side effects such as internal hemorrhage and stroke.

Once stabilized, doctors may offer patients a procedure called an angioplasty. This is a mechanical method of expanding the diameter of a blocked coronary artery, thereby increasing blood flow to the heart. This is done by inserting a thin, balloon-tipped tube into the obstructed artery and then inflating the balloon, which pushes the plaque open and improves the diameter of the vessel. Sometimes, a stent is left in place in an effort to keep the vessel wide open.

Although this sounds like an ingeniously simple idea, there can be severe complications, such as tearing the vessel. Another complication is an embolism, which occurs when the plaque is fragmented as a side effect of the procedure. Pieces of the plaque then travel through the bloodstream until they lodge in smaller vessels. If they end up in the circulation of the brain, they can cause a stroke. Your doctor would discuss these risks with you before the angioplasty.

Occasionally, bypass surgery may be needed, sometimes urgently. In this surgery, the obstruction is bypassed by taking a nonessential vein from another part of the body (usually the leg) and inserting it onto the coronary (heart) artery so that blood will flow around the blockage— similar to creating a traffic detour. Coronary bypass surgery produces an immediate improvement in the oxygenation of the heart, but it should be viewed as only a temporary solution. Unless you take measures to correct the underlying cause of atherosclerosis and chronic inflammation, the new "detour" will most likely become clogged with inflamed plaque. If that happens, the symptoms will recur.

Prevention of Heart Attack

Ideally, the best course of action is to prevent a heart attack in the first place. By preventing the first assault on the heart, you may also be able to prevent subsequent cardiac arrhythmias and heart failure. Because there is no one single cause of heart disease, preventing its onset requires a multipronged approach. In the past, a great deal of attention was paid to lowering cholesterol levels using both dietary and pharmacologic interventions. Interestingly, most heart attacks happen in people who have normal cholesterol levels.[2] The more recent and more effective approach is to decrease chronic inflammation within the body. It is inflammation of the fibrous covering of the plaque that renders it vulnerable to rupture, leading to subsequent formation of blood clots (thrombi) within the heart's blood vessels. This is why the prevention of coronary artery disease requires methods that incorporate anti-inflammatory, antithrombotic, and antioxidant techniques. It is also useful to reduce the amount of cholesterol contained in low-density lipoproteins known as LDL-C[3], shifting the balance of cholesterol subtypes to a more favorable ratio.

Sleep

Follow the previously mentioned guidelines to optimize the quality of your sleep. Strive to sleep at least seven hours each night.

---

2. G. A. Plotnikoff et al., "Prevention of Atherosclerosis," in *Integrative Medicine*, ed. David Rakel, 1st ed. (Philadelphia: Saunders, 2003), 559–571.

3. Plotnikoff et al., "Prevention of Atherosclerosis," 559–571.

Anti-inflammatories

Using food to decrease the amount of chronic inflammation within your body is probably the easiest and most efficient way to create a healthier cardiovascular system. One component of our diet that can affect inflammation is fatty acids. Fatty acids are exactly that—organic acids that occur naturally as fats or oils. This may sound like something you wouldn't want in your body, but fatty acids are the essential building blocks of hormones and are involved in gene expression and immune function. Also, fatty acids are found in the membranes of every cell in your body, particularly your brain and nervous system.

There are various types of fatty acids, but the two that humans cannot synthesize in our bodies are omega-6 and omega-3. For this reason they are called essential fatty acids, because we must get them from our food. The ratio of omega-6 to omega-3 fatty acids in our bodies can greatly influence our health. Omega-6 fatty acids generate more inflammatory mediators than omega-3 fatty acids; this is not such a terrible thing if the balance of the two is correct. However, our modern diet has seen staggering changes in the last fifty years, particularly in the area of omega-6 to omega-3 ratios: the balance has shifted, with catastrophic results. Scientists have demonstrated that this dietary disequilibrium directly contributes to the development of cardiovascular disease as well as most chronic illnesses known to Western societies such as cancer, arthritis, and autoimmune conditions.[4]

To increase your intake of omega-3 fatty acids, you can eat cold-water fish twice a week. Such fish include wild-caught mackerel, salmon, albacore tuna, and sardines. Farm-raised fish may have been fed cereal-based food, whereas wild-caught fish eat algae, which is much higher in omega-3 fatty acids. For this reason, wild-caught is a better choice if it is available to you. If not, farm-raised cold-water fish still has many benefits and you should incorporate it into your diet if wild-caught is not accessible.

---

4. D. Rakel, "The Anti-Inflammatory Diet," in *Integrative Medicine*, ed. David Rakel, 1st ed. (Philadelphia: Saunders, 2003), 667–671.

Aside from fish, omega-3 fatty acids can be found in abundance in flax seed, soybeans, green leafy vegetables like kale and chard, and nuts, especially walnuts.

Taking a supplement rich in omega-3 fatty acids, in the form of fish oils or flaxseed oil, is another way to help prevent heart disease. A sufficient amount would be 1 gram/day in addition to various antioxidants described in the next section.[5] If you are actively treating heart disease or other inflammatory conditions, the amount of omega-3 fatty acids required can be considerably higher, but you should consult your physician before increasing the dose.

Antioxidants

Oxidation is a process that occurs within the body as a consequence of normal metabolic activities. You have observed oxidation at work in the outside world if you have ever seen a fruit turn brown after it is cut open or seen metal rust. Oxidation within the body creates a type of molecule called a free radical. Free radicals are unstable and attach to themselves and other compounds. They have received a lot of bad publicity in recent years, being associated with the creation of genetic mutations that can lead to cancer and other degenerative diseases. But the truth is, free radicals are essential to life. They are the intermediate steps in chemical reactions that assist your immune system in controlling infection. Free radicals are also involved in cell signaling and regulate such processes as dilating or constricting blood vessels to influence blood pressure.

To prevent the presence of excessive amounts of free radicals, you can increase your intake of antioxidants, either with food and/or with dietary supplements. Fruits, vegetables, legumes, and whole grains are excellent sources of natural antioxidants. Various population-based studies have demonstrated that people whose diets are centered on these foods have less heart disease and fewer cardiovascular-related deaths.[6]

---

5. Rakel, "Anti-Inflammatory Diet," 667–671.

6. M. de Lorgeril et al., "Mediterranean Diet, Traditional Risk Factors, and the Rate of Cardiovascular Complications after Myocardial Infarction: Final Report of the Lyon Diet Heart Study," *Circulation* 99 (6): 779–785.

Vitamins

Beyond food, certain supplements may be suggested by your doctor for their benefit as antioxidants. These include vitamins such as B6, B12, and folic acid. In the past, these B vitamins were recommended in hope of preventing heart disease because they decrease levels of homocysteine in the blood. Homocysteine is an amino acid that may be involved in long-term damage to the blood vessel lining, leading to plaque formation. The reasoning was sound, but well-designed studies have failed to find a causal link between elevated homocysteine levels and heart disease. Put another way, although B vitamins have been shown in observational studies to lower homocysteine levels, there does not seem to be a concurrent decrease in heart disease.[7]

Vitamin D may also be recommended. Receptors for vitamin D are found in heart muscle cells and the walls of the arteries. There is a known association between low vitamin D levels and coronary artery disease (as well as some cancers) but the mechanism is not quite clear. It is recommended that vitamin D be used as a supplement to raise blood levels above 30 ng/ml, which is the lower limit of the normal range.[8] The dosing for vitamin D falls between 1,000 and 5,000 IU per day, depending on the degree of deficiency.

Other Supplements

Coenzyme Q_{10} (also known as CoQ_{10} or ubiquinol) is a vitamin-like molecule that is intricately involved in energy production in our cells and also acts as a free radical scavenger with potent antioxidant properties. Coenzyme Q_{10} inhibits the oxidation of LDL and other substances, decreasing inflammation within your bloodstream. You can find coenzyme Q_{10} in eggs and beef as well as spinach, grains, and legumes. If

---

7. Chi Zhang et al., "Association between B Vitamins Supplementation and Risk of Cardiovascular Outcomes: A Cumulative Meta-Analysis of Randomized Controlled Trials," *PLoS One* 9 (9): e107060, doi:10.1371/journal.pone.0107060.

8. Stephen Devries, "Coronary Artery Disease," in *Integrative Medicine*, ed. David Rakel, 4th ed. (Philadelphia: Elsevier, 2018), 260.

you are taking a cholesterol-lowering medication, you would need to take a larger amount of coenzyme Q_{10} because these sorts of drugs deplete CoQ_{10} levels. The recommended dose is coenzyme Q_{10}, 200 mcg daily, or 400 mcg daily if taking cholesterol-lowering drugs.

Antithrombotics

Taking antioxidant and anti-inflammatory supplements and eating foods that will prevent inflammation of intravascular plaque is very beneficial, but it is also important to reduce the chance of blood clot (thrombus) formation within the vessels. Antithrombotic activity can be increased by food, supplements, and medications.

Garlic and onions both are noted for their anti-platelet activity and their ability to help break down clots that have already formed. Botanical supplements such as ginseng, hawthorn, and gingko all have anti-platelet effects that can help increase blood flow; however, they may also cause unwanted bleeding. Before taking any of these botanicals, it is imperative that you speak to your doctor to ensure these supplements will not adversely interact with any of your medications and that they are appropriate for your condition. As ginseng, hawthorn, and gingko are commonly used in Chinese herbal formulas for cardiovascular problems, you must also be sure to discuss all supplements and medications that you are taking with your practitioner of Eastern medicine.

Another supplement that inhibits platelet clumping is magnesium. People who have low blood levels of magnesium are at greater risk of experiencing a blood clot initiated by platelet aggregation. Additionally, patients with coronary artery disease (CAD) can decrease their risk of a platelet-dependent blood clot by 35 percent if they add magnesium to their daily supplements. This reduction in risk was evident even when these patients were already taking aspirin. Aspirin is a standard medication used to prevent blood clots in the heart or brain of people who have underlying risk factors for such an event, such as hypertension, CAD, or prior heart attack or stroke. Because of the risk of bleeding from the stomach lining, the risks and benefits of daily aspirin ingestion should be discussed with your physician before starting such a regimen.

Cholesterol-Lowering Strategies

The role of cholesterol in the development of coronary artery disease seems to be controversial. As mentioned above, it may be that inflammation is a greater threat to your cardiovascular health than is cholesterol. Everyone needs cholesterol because it is a precursor to many biochemical compounds that are essential to life. The fact that 50 percent of those who suffer heart attacks have normal standard cholesterol profiles indicates that there is more to coronary artery disease than simply cholesterol.

In fact, closer study shows that there are even more subtypes of low-density lipoproteins (LDL) and high-density lipoproteins than was previously thought. When the link between elevated cholesterol and heart disease was first established, it was soon determined that ratios between LDL, HDL, and triglycerides were also important influences on the progression of coronary artery disease. Now, further investigations have yielded greater insight into lipid metabolism, and subtypes of subtypes have been discovered.

At least seven subtypes of LDL and five subtypes of HDL have been detected. It appears that some of the LDL subtypes are more detrimental to health than others and that some of the HDL subtypes are more beneficial than others. The ratio of subtypes within each category may be more significant than levels of LDL or HDL overall. These subtype ratios can be affected by diet and supplements. This would explain why some populations who have very high levels of cholesterol have very little actual cardiovascular illness. To have your cholesterol subtype levels checked, you could ask your doctor to request an advanced lipid profile.[9]

That being said, there are definitely changes you can make in your diet and supplement regimen that can lower your cholesterol levels. These

---

9. "Advanced Lipid Profile Testing," www.scrippsintegrativemedicine.org/lifestyl/test.htm, accessed March 13, 2013.

include decreasing your intake of saturated fats like those found in red meat and dairy products and increasing your intake of soy, oat bran, and psyllium (a source of soluble fiber), all of which have been shown to lower LDL levels.

Lifestyle Interventions

Aside from a biochemical approach to decreasing the risk of cardiovascular disease, Western scientists have been investigating the various ways in which lifestyle changes can influence heart health. Exercise is a well-established intervention that can lower the risk of myocardial infarction as well as many other diseases, including diabetes, hypertension, and cancer. Interestingly, at least with respect to cardiovascular disease, exercise intensity did not matter as much as frequency and consistency.[10]

In recent years, the allopathic medical community has acknowledged the importance that psychological and social stressors have upon coronary artery disease. This realization has led to studies that investigate how relieving these stressors can decrease the risk of cardiovascular morbidity and mortality. In many people who experience chronic or acute stress, anxiety, or depression, certain physiologic changes occur within the nervous system and influence all aspects of the body,[11] including the hormonal, immunologic, and cardiovascular systems. Interventions that have been shown to decrease stress, anxiety, and depression include meditation, yoga, biofeedback, tai chi, and qigong. All these modalities have been used to decrease the risk of myocardial infarction in susceptible individuals. Also, in patients who have already had a heart attack, such mind-body healing interventions can prevent re-infarction.[12]

---

10. Russell Greenfield, "Heart Failure," in *Integrative Medicine*, ed. David Rakel, 4th ed. (Philadelphia: Elsevier, 2018), 254.

11. S. V. Arnold et al., "Perceived Stress in Myocardial Infarction: Long-Term Mortality and Health Status Outcomes," *Journal of the American College of Cardiology* 60 (18): 1756–1763.

12. C. L. Chan et al., "A Systematic Review of the Effectiveness of Qigong Exercise in Cardiac Rehabilitation," *American Journal of Chinese Medicine* 40 (2): 255–267; A. Dalusung-Angosta, "The Impact of Tai Chi Exercise on Coronary Heart Disease: A

Specific qigong exercises that can benefit your heart are discussed in detail in chapter 4.

Summary of Western Interventions in the Prevention of Heart Attack

These interventions can be used after discussion with your health-care provider. Your physician can help you determine which recommendations are the best for your particular situation.

Sleep

Strive for at least seven hours of restorative sleep in a twenty-four-hour period

Nutrition

Include six to nine servings of fruits and vegetables daily

> Soy protein
>
> Oat bran
>
> Cold-water, wild-caught fish
>
> Flaxseed
>
> Walnuts
>
> Garlic
>
> Onions

Avoid saturated fats

Supplements

Niacin: up to 1,500 mg twice daily (check cholesterol and liver function after six weeks of this therapy)

Coenzyme Q_{10}: 200 mcg daily (400 mcg in patients taking HMG CoA reductase inhibitors to lower cholesterol)

Vitamin D: 1,000–5,000 IU daily, sufficient to raise blood levels above 30 ng/ml

Flaxseed oil or fish oil: 4–16 g daily

Systematic Review," *Journal of the American Academy of Nurse Practitioners* 23 (7): 376–381.

Medications (with your doctor's prescription)
  Enteric-coated aspirin: 81–325 mg daily
  Cholesterol-lowering drugs

Lifestyle interventions
  Achieve your ideal body weight
  Perform aerobic exercise on most days of the week
  Reduce stress by incorporating any of these mind-body modalities
    meditation
    tai chi
    qigong
    yoga
    biofeedback
    support of family, friends, or formal support groups

Arrhythmias

Another form of heart disease is an abnormal heart rate, known as an arrhythmia. Arrhythmias occur as a consequence of abnormal electrical activity in the cardiac conduction pathways. Usually, one area is the natural pacemaker. There can be many causes of abnormal electrical conduction in the heart: aside from heart attacks, other causes include imbalances in blood chemistry, side effects of medications, and disturbances in the nervous system that controls the heart. If the heart beats too slowly, certain cells in the heart will cause the rate to increase as a sort of fail-safe mechanism. These are called "ectopic" beats, meaning that the electrical activity arises from a part of the heart that is not normally involved in this process.

The heart is a pump. The rate at which the heart contracts depends on electrical signaling; this signaling can be too fast, too slow, or irregular. A common symptom of an arrhythmia is palpitations, or the sensation that your heart is pounding. Sometimes, the arrhythmia is very short-lived, and the patient experiences the sensation of chest palpitations for only a few seconds or minutes. Sometimes, it lasts longer—even hours. If the arrhythmia prevents the heart from moving blood efficiently, all parts of the body, including the heart, will not receive enough oxygen, which can result in dizziness, fainting, chest pain, heart attack, and possibly death. Blood clots can form within the chambers of the heart because of the irregular blood flow. Such blood clots sometimes get pumped out of the heart and end up in the brain, causing a stroke. To decrease the risk of this serious complication, your cardiologist would prescribe blood-thinners. Usually, though, most arrhythmias are not life-threatening.

Treatment of Arrhythmias

A physician should perform the initial evaluation of cardiac arrhythmias, and if your symptoms are serious, you should be seen by a cardiologist. It is important to determine the cause and rule out any dangerous underlying problem. If you feel that your heart is racing and it does not slow down on its own after a few moments, or if it is beating so slowly that you are becoming weak and dizzy, you should seek medical attention. Your heart may not be able to pump enough blood to maintain your blood pressure or oxygenate your heart or brain. Acute management of an arrhythmia in an emergency room setting can include various medications or even a procedure called cardioversion. With this method, a measured electrical shock is applied to the chest wall. If successful, this will essentially reset the heart's natural electrical pacer and a normal rate and rhythm will return.

The treatment of an arrhythmia is quite complex and depends entirely on its source and triggers. Investigations include checking blood biochemistry and undergoing an electrocardiogram (EKG), which examines the electrical output of the heart, and a cardiac echo, which is an ultrasound of the heart that looks at its structure and blood flow within the chambers. Often, an arrhythmia is not captured on an EKG, and it is necessary to wear a heart monitor for twenty-four hours or more to detect an abnormality. If you are taking any medications that can alter the heart rate, blood tests can be performed to determine whether your drug levels are too high or too low. If your medication levels were not correct, your dose would be adjusted. If imbalances of minerals within the blood were found, they would need to be corrected. For example, arrhythmias can be caused by either too much or too little potassium, magnesium, or calcium.

The majority of arrhythmias are not serious. However, if an arrhythmia is life-threatening and causes changes in heart function or blood pressure, it will require specialized interventions. These may include an artificial pacemaker, which speeds up the heart; an implanted defibrillator, which can restart the heart in the case of sudden cardiac arrest; or radiofrequency ablation. Radiofrequency ablation is a technique used when a small area of the heart is beating independently from the normal electrical system, called an ectopic focus. Radiofrequency ablation will destroy that small area of the heart to allow the natural pacemaker to take precedence.

Once an arrhythmia has been determined to be relatively benign, you and your physician can establish what sort of treatment will best relieve your symptoms. Medications may be called for to either speed up or slow down your heart rate. These different medications are specific for the type of cardiac arrhythmia in question. You should also let your doctor know if you are taking any supplements that contain ephedra or gingko biloba, as it is possible that these botanicals can trigger heart rate abnormalities.

Sometimes, lifestyle choices can influence the heart rate, such as excessive intake of caffeine, tobacco use, and alcohol consumption. Even chocolate could be the culprit! Large or fatty meals that distend the stomach can activate one of the nerves (vagus nerve) that has a role in slowing the heart. This can result in palpitations or fainting. You could experiment with adjusting the size of your meals or eliminating your intake of the above substances to see whether it makes any difference to your symptoms.

Exercise can be used to decrease cardiac arrhythmias, but *not* by those whose abnormality is considered life-threatening. If your arrhythmia is triggered by stress or anxiety, exercise can be very beneficial. It may seem counterintuitive that stress-induced arrhythmias can be improved by exercise, but being stressed or anxious causes an increase in the flight-or-fight response generated by the release of chemicals called catecholamines (adrenaline) by your sympathetic nervous system. This involuntary response raises your heart rate and blood pressure. It is balanced by the parasympathetic nervous system, of which the vagus nerve is a part. The parasympathetic nervous system lowers your heart rate and blood pressure. Exercise decreases your sensitivity to catecholamines (adrenaline) and drops the actual level of these substances in your body. Exercise also dampens the activity of the sympathetic nervous system and increases that of the vagus nerve (parasympathetic nervous system). As a result, you should experience less severe palpitations, along with a greater sense of calm.

Another way to maintain a healthy balance between the sympathetic and parasympathetic nervous systems is to incorporate mind-body techniques into your treatment plan. Examples of these modalities include biofeedback, meditation, relaxation techniques, qigong, and tai chi. These are discussed in greater detail in the discussion of the Eastern approach to treating heart disease. Acupuncture can also be used to decrease the intensity and frequency of these episodes. It has been demonstrated in Western studies that certain arrhythmias respond well to acupuncture treatments as well as to Chinese herbal formulas.[13]

In addition to Chinese herbs, other Western botanicals have been used as anti-arrhythmics and, in fact, form the basis of several cardiac medications prescribed for this purpose. For example, digoxin is derived from foxglove and quinidine from cinchona bark; both are anti-arrhythmic medications.

---

13. M. Deng et al., "Clinical Observation on the Treatment of Atrial Fibrillation with Amiodarone Combined with Shenmai Injection," *Chinese Journal of Integrative Medicine* 16 (5): 453–456; F. Lombardi et al., "Acupuncture for Paroxysmal and Persistent Atrial Fibrillation: An Effective Non-Pharmacological Tool?" *World Journal of Cardiology* 4 (3): 60–65; A. Lomuscio et al., "Efficacy of Acupuncture in Preventing Atrial Fibrillation Recurrences after Electrical Cardioversion," *Journal of Cardiovascular Electrophysiology* 22 (3): 241–247.

Vitamins and minerals can also assist in controlling an abnormal heart rate. Calcium, magnesium, selenium, potassium, coenzyme Q_{10}, and vitamin C have all proven useful in a variety of studies.[14]

Omega-3 fatty acids have been found to decrease episodes of certain arrhythmias and also decrease the risk for sudden death caused by arrhythmia. In a study that involved more than 11,000 patients who had had a heart attack in the previous three months, those who were given fish oil (an excellent source of omega-3 fatty acids) dropped their risk of arrhythmia-induced sudden death by half.[15]

Whichever medication, procedure, supplement, or lifestyle change you use to control your cardiac arrhythmia, the goal is to decrease your symptoms without unduly increasing your risk of side effects.

Heart Valve Disease

Disease of the heart valves can have many causes, including infection, genetic disorders, trauma, tumors, and malformations. The valves are located between the heart chambers or between chambers and large blood vessels. If they don't close properly, either too little blood will be moving forward (because the valve doesn't open enough and restricts the amount of blood that can pass through with each heartbeat) or the blood will back up in the heart chambers (because the valve never completely closes between heartbeats, and backward blood flow occurs). Sometimes, the blood can back up into the lungs, making it difficult to breathe. In either case, long-term damage to heart muscle can occur, causing heart chamber enlargement, cardiac arrhythmias, and congestive heart failure.

Valvular Disease

If the valvular problem is only minor, the usual management is simply observation over time to ensure there is no worsening of the situation. If the abnormal flow within the heart is severe enough, causing significant

---

14. Brian Olshansky, "Arrhythmias," in *Integrative Medicine*, ed. David Rakel, 1st ed. (Philadelphia: Saunders, 2003), 195–206.

15. Olshansky, "Arrhythmias," 195–206.

symptoms and disabilities, the offending valve may need to be replaced. In the past, the only way to replace a valve was through open-heart surgery. These days there are more options. By using small incisions, video or robotic-assisted valve replacement can be used. These minimally invasive procedures cause much less trauma to the chest wall than do open-heart procedures. Even less invasive are transcatheter valve replacements. It is now possible, under certain circumstances, to replace a heart valve through a catheter that is threaded through the large blood vessels at the groin. Initially, only the aortic valve was replaced in this manner, but now it is possible to replace a mitral valve with a transcatheter procedure.

Whichever route your surgeon recommends, the goal is to remove the defective valve and replace it with either a mechanical valve or a valve from biological tissue. Having a mechanical valve requires being on lifelong blood thinners to prevent blood clots from forming on the valve, leading to further complications. Biological tissue includes heart valves from human donors and porcine or bovine valves or similarly strong tissue, called pericardium, from these animals. The advantage of a biological valve is that blood thinners are not required.

The choice of procedure and type of valve is a complex decision that is best discussed with a cardiovascular surgeon.

Heart Failure

All types of cardiovascular disease, if left untreated, have the potential to lead to heart failure. This condition is exactly what it sounds like: the heart becomes so damaged that it cannot efficiently pump blood to the lungs and/or other organs of the body. As with almost all chronic conditions, the very best treatment for heart failure is to prevent it in the first place. Once established, heart failure is very difficult to treat.

Looking at heart failure from an individual's point of view, this illness brings with it potentially progressively debilitating symptoms such as shortness of breath, fatigue, heart palpitations, and swollen feet and legs. Depending on the degree and type of heart failure, some people experience these symptoms with very mild exertion or even while at rest.

Examining heart failure from a societal perspective, the statistics are staggering. In the United States, starting at age forty, the lifetime risk of developing heart failure is 20 percent.[16] With advancing age, this statistic increases. More than 50 percent of those who develop heart disease will die within five years from the time they are diagnosed.[17]

As the population ages, the absolute number of people with heart failure will rise. Already more than 5.7 million Americans suffer with heart failure. The costs of managing this condition—both the direct cost of treatment and the indirect cost of lost productivity for these individuals—was estimated in 2010 at more than $39 billion. This number will escalate over time.[18]

Diseases that would put you at risk for heart failure are hypertension, heart attack, severe lung disease, sleep apnea, diabetes, obesity, and mood disorders. This last risk factor again highlights the connection between emotions and heart health. It has been seen that depression is an independent risk factor for the development of heart failure. In fact, in some studies, depression increased this risk by as much as 40 percent, compared with people who do not suffer from depression but had similar health profiles as the study group in every other respect.[19]

In chapter 2, we discussed the normal cardiac circulation and looked at how the heart sends blood from the right-sided chambers to the lungs for oxygenation and the release of carbon dioxide, a product of cellular metabolism. The oxygenated blood is then pushed through the lungs by the force generated by the heart and, via the pulmonary veins, arrives at the left side of the heart to be pumped out to the rest of the body, as well as to the cardiac vessels that nourish the heart itself. The heart's ability to circulate blood can be diminished for many reasons, but the common

---

16. Russell Greenfield, "Heart Failure," in *Integrative Medicine*, ed. David Rakel, 4th ed. (Philadelphia: Elsevier, 2018), 242.

17. Centers for Disease Control, "Heart Failure Fact Sheet," https://www.cdc.gov/dhdsp/data_statistics/fact_sheets/fs_heart_failure.htm, accessed July 30, 2019.

18. Russell Greenfield, "Heart Failure," in *Integrative Medicine*, ed. David Rakel, 4th ed. (Philadelphia: Elsevier, 2018), 242.

19. Greenfield, "Heart Failure," 250.

result is that the heart cannot keep up with the demands of the body. Let's take a brief look at how different conditions can lead to heart failure.

High blood pressure (hypertension) forces the left side of the heart to work harder to overcome the increased pressure of narrower and less flexible blood vessels. Imagine having to increase the water flow in a garden hose to overcome an obstruction farther down the line. Over time, this increased load causes the heart chambers to dilate and the muscle walls to thicken, which, eventually, decreases the amount of blood the heart can pump out with each heartbeat. The percentage of blood within the left ventricle that leaves the heart with every beat is known as the ejection fraction. A normal ejection fraction is about 50–70 percent. As the ejection fraction gets lower, people start to experience symptoms such as fatigue and shortness of breath. Because the amount of blood is smaller within each heartbeat, the heart starts to compensate by beating faster in order to distribute more blood during the same amount of time. This increased heart rate puts additional strain on the heart. You can see how this can become a vicious downward cycle.

If a person has suffered a heart attack, the muscle of the heart may be permanently damaged, decreasing the efficiency with which the heart can circulate blood. Abnormal heart valves can leak and cause a backup of blood within the system and a decrease in the amount of oxygenated blood that can leave the heart to nourish all the organs and cells of the body.

Severe lung disease can create increased pressure in the pulmonary circulation and lead to a backup of blood in the right side of the heart. This can cause the wall of the right ventricle to thicken and even cause blood and its fluid component to back up into the veins of the abdomen and the legs. This is one reason that people may experience swollen feet and ankles.

Treatment of Heart Failure

Heart failure, once it has begun, is extraordinarily difficult to treat. The best treatment is prevention. Physicians will aggressively treat all the conditions that can lead to heart failure, including hypertension, coronary artery disease, diabetes, mood disorders, and obesity. Obesity, in and of itself, incurs a 10 percent risk of heart failure even in the absence of other known risk factors, through a process called lipid cardiotoxicity, in which adipocytes (fat cells) are deposited between heart muscle cells and prevent optimal contractility.[20]

The goal of treatment is to minimize symptoms and optimize cardiac function. Therefore the treatment protocols chosen depend on the cause. Patients with heart failure should be cared for by a cardiologist. Anything that exacerbates the underlying cause of heart failure should be eliminated if possible. Even some commonly used medications can cause heart failure, such as ibuprofen and naproxen, and older types of blood pressure medication called calcium channel blockers. Medications are the mainstay of treatment, but quality of life can be greatly enhanced by improving a patient's nutrition with an anti-inflammatory or Mediterranean-type diet, decreased fluid and salt intake, stress management techniques, and restorative sleep. Even exercise tolerance can be improved and should be undertaken in a certified cardiac rehabilitation program. Spiritual needs should be attended to, and pastoral care services used as requested.

Cardiac medications are generally used in combinations to control blood pressure and heart rate as well as blood volume. One medication used particularly in heart failure is digitalis; also known as digoxin, digitalis is extracted from the foxglove plant. It is used to strengthen the contractions of the heart so it can pump more efficiently.

Other ways to improve the strength and rate of the heartbeat are through the use of biomechanical devices. Some patients see significant improvement in the quality and length of life with the use of special pacemakers that correct ventricular arrhythmias. These devices may also

---

20. Imo A. Ebong, "Mechanisms of Heart Failure in Obesity," *Obesity Research Clinical Practice* 8 (6): e540–e548, doi:10.1016/j.orcp.2013.12.005.

include a cardioverter defibrillator that administers a shock of electricity if the heart stops beating for too long.[21]

Whereas cardioverter defibrillators use the electrical system of the heart to modify its beat, other inventions, called ventricular assist devices (VAD), mechanically pump blood from the heart to vessels. The most common type is a left ventricular device (LVAD), though the right ventricle or even both ventricles can be assisted in this manner. In the case of the LVAD, the blood leaves the left ventricle into the device, which is attached to both the ventricle and the aorta. The pump is placed along the conduit between the left ventricle and the aorta. Early versions of this device used a pulsatile pump, but now an impeller is used to push a continuous flow of blood into circulation. One interesting consequence of the continuous flow is that the patient may not have a pulse. Ventricular assist devices can be used as a "bridge," keeping a patient alive until a donor heart is available for transplant, but some people simply live out their lives with these devices in place, sometimes for years.

Before we move on to discuss the Eastern approach to heart disease, it is worth reiterating that the absolute best way to treat heart failure is to prevent it. Do everything you can to keep your heart healthy!

Eastern Approach to Preventing and Healing Heart Disease

The purpose of the practice of qigong, tai chi, and Eastern medicine in general is to bring balance to the body's energetic system, which is connected to our emotions, organ function, metabolic processes, muscle resilience, joint flexibility, equilibrium, and immune functions. These practices improve the function of all these systems and decrease inflammation. Eastern medicine emphasizes a holistic approach to bringing balance and harmony to the mind-body. Treatments include herbs, diet changes, self-care, cultivating a healthy mind disposition, and physical

---

21. Russell Greenfield, "Heart Failure," in *Integrative Medicine*, ed. David Rakel, 4th ed. (Philadelphia: Elsevier, 2018), 242–250.

training such as tai chi and qigong. The practice helps stabilize your body and manage the effects of stress. It is the mind-body philosophy that is the key to its effectiveness.

When we are exposed to a traumatic event or a perceived threat, our adrenaline suddenly increases, our heart rate increases, and our blood pressure elevates. Our blood cortisol level increases, and that causes our blood sugar to rise—this is our natural alarm system. Our body and brain communicate to control our behavior and mood. Once a perceived threat has passed, hormone levels return to normal. As adrenaline and cortisol levels drop, the heart rate and blood pressure return to baseline levels and other systems resume their regular activities.

If a person carries chronic stress, his elevated hormone levels continue to stay in the blood, which can have adverse effects. The adrenaline continues to constrict blood vessels and can cause chronically elevated blood pressure. Eventually the blood vessels in the heart will constrict. The cortisol will continue to increase blood sugar, decrease immune system function, and weaken the muscles in the body. This long-term activation of the stress-response system can disrupt almost all of the body's processes, create an internal environment of chronic inflammation, and put the body at great risk for numerous health problems.

Prevention is a lifestyle. Being able to control our own lives is so important for maintaining our quality of life. We can discover ways to make choices that lead us toward better health. We are often influenced by commercials, political decisions, religions, and peer pressure. We allow others to control our lives and behaviors; we want to dress like others, do our hair like others, buy things like others, and we don't want others to laugh at us, or look down on us. We may feel that becoming rich can lead to happiness. My question is, why do we allow others to control our lives? Do we have an identity? Do we have character? Do we know who we are? If we ask these questions and are able to answer them honestly, we may feel differently. I don't want others to control my life; I like myself and I have my own special character; I am smart, and I know what I want and what I don't want. If someone ridicules me, I know they have a problem. No matter what they say, I am still a good person, a smart person, I have my strengths and I no longer allow them to get on my case or determine who I am. By affirming these things, we feel good and strong about ourselves. By feeling strong and confident, our stress level is reduced; from reduced stress in life, our health improves.

In 2011, when I was working in my Boston office, a patient asked me, "Why do we live?" For many years I was able to answer pretty much every patient's question, but this time I was stumped. I did not know what to say or how to reply to this question. To save my face, I had to say something, so I said, "Well, God made us to live, we live." Later I regretted saying this. I realized I did not answer his question.

This patient had had a heart attack the year before and went through surgery. He was not well after surgery. He had fatigue, depression, anxiety, insomnia, muscle pain, and trouble focusing. He had chronic stress, and chronic stress is one of the biggest causes of heart disease and hypertension. Even though he had bypass surgery, his chronic stress was still the biggest obstacle to his healing. I realized that his medication alone could not help his stress; therefore I prescribed a type of qigong I named Therapeutic Qi Gong. I recommended he get the DVD of this qigong form and asked him to practice it at least four times a week.

In several weeks, he felt better and calmer, he felt less stress, and he had more energy. I explained to him that it was not a quick cure but a healing journey that he should practice for a lifetime.

Natural Healing Modalities for Prevention or Rehabilitation of Heart Disease

In natural healing, there are always multiple approaches. There is no single approach for all, and it is not a magic pill. Think about the body. It contains many parts, and every part has its function and needs to be cared for. Many people are frustrated with their medical professionals. What we need to understand is that conventional medicine is not designed for healing. It is designed for saving lives in emergency situations and symptom relief in chronic conditions. Healing is different. Healing is a mind-set and a process. A quality daily practice will make the difference in your life.

Quality practice includes

- Stress management
- Dietary changes
- Herbal medicine and nutritional support
- Acupuncture/tui na treatment
- Qigong or tai chi practice
- Mindful meditation
- Daoist learning and practice

Stress Management

Stress is the reaction of our mind and body in response to something that does not go smoothly. We can learn how to manage the effects of stress. We practice not allowing the stressor to affect our emotions. Doing so helps us keep our mind clear, focused, and calm.

Qigong, tai chi, meditation, deep breaths, and other exercises that strengthen our body and balance our mind provide tools for a logical, healthy way to deal with life stress. Other helpful things to do are listening to music, engaging in hobbies, fostering healthy friendships, participating in outdoor activities, reading, traveling, watching comedy TV shows or movies, or playing sports. By doing these things, we can avoid carrying negative feelings when stressful situations happen to us.

I often tell my qigong and tai chi students, "Practice to build strong qi. We call qi the defense that can protect us from negative energy toward us." Many of my students tell me they are able to block negative energy and they are better able to deal with stressors. If we hold on to negative feelings, we create chronic stress, and we harm ourselves chronically. Eventually we become sick or create an imbalance in the organ system.

Do not be embarrassed to get professional assistance, either Western or Eastern. For the Western approach, you can get some counseling. The Eastern approach includes acupuncture treatments, or a good therapeutic massage. Tui na (Chinese therapeutic massage) is very effective because it works on the body meridian pathways to removes blockages.

Genetic factors can affect a person's ability to deal with stress. Life experience is another factor, and some reactions to stress can be traced to a traumatic event in the past. Everyone has different levels of dealing with stress, and some people deal better than others. But no matter what the reason, following the above recommendations can help you a great deal with stress management.

Dietary Changes

Changing your diet can change your health and life. There are many books and articles talking about diet, and sometimes the information can be confusing because there are so many different opinions. For heart disease or hypertension, some general principles about diet apply. People who have heart disease should avoid too much meat, dairy, fat, junk food, butter, cheese, ice cream, and sweets. For more explicit instructions about how to adopt an anti-inflammatory diet, please see the True Wellness Checklist in chapter 6. Even without specific recommendations, you can get a good idea whether your diet is balanced just by looking at the proportions of the types of food on your plate. Imagine that your plate is a pie graph and a full plate has a volume of 100 percent. An appropriate diet should be made up of 50 percent vegetables; 10 to 20 percent meat or other protein foods; 20 to 30 percent legumes, brown rice, soy, nuts and seeds, or other whole grains; and 10 percent other.

This way of eating is very simple: low calorie, low fat, high fiber. It can help prevent other illnesses and conditions such as diabetes, obesity, high cholesterol, and hypertension. But it is not black and white, because each person is different. We have different levels of activities, jobs, and eating habits, different metabolisms, and different body sizes.

Proper hydration is an important and often forgotten element of diet. It is essential in helping to cope with stress. I have seen a connection between dehydration and patients who have poor stress management skills. Dehydration affects the brain and diminishes logical thinking. A general rule is to drink 64 ounces of water per day. Of course, that amount will vary from person to person. Many factors influence how much water you should consume. Some factors include your age, physical activity, and the temperature of your environment. Thirst may not be the best indicator of dehydration. In fact, by the time you are thirsty, your blood volume has already decreased because of a lack of fluids. Other symptoms that may occur earlier than thirst include dark urine, headache, fatigue, and even confusion, especially in the elderly.

Herbal Medicine and Nutritional Support

Herbal medicine in China is very popular. Herbs are now available in pill form, which is becoming more popular because of its convenience. In the United States, practitioners of Eastern medicine prescribe herbal formulas that complement their treatment and help achieve healing results. To maintain optimal health, patients also need to incorporate nutritional support into their daily lives. For many years I was against supplemental nutrition because I believed we could get enough nutrition from foods. I was wrong. Our foods are losing nutrition thanks to the commercial food industry and GMOs. Also, our bodies don't get enough nutrition because we are too busy to eat well. In many cases, heart disease is caused by and/or accelerated by stress and poor diet.

The right nutritional supplements are important for healing and prevention. These recommendations are similar to the list recommended for the Western approach to heart disease and include fish oil with omega-3, CoQ_{10}, vitamin D, and hawthorn berry extract. You can find dosing instructions in the section above titled Summary of Western Interventions in the Prevention of Heart Attack.

Acupuncture/Tui Na Treatment

The combination of Eastern and Western medicine leads to optimal healing results. The two modalities complement each other and promote symptomatic relief, open blocked arteries, and prevent relapses.

How does acupuncture work in assisting healing? First, acupuncture treatment relaxes the person and removes the body tension. It relaxes the whole body and brain and relieves tension in the muscular system and vascular system. The relaxation of the body, mind, and blood vessels allows the blood to flow to all parts of the body including the heart. If your blood vessels are relaxed, your blood pressure drops naturally (if you have hypertension). Certain acupuncture points are known to strengthen the contractility of the heart and even regulate cardiac arrhythmias. In Eastern medicine, we understand that an arrhythmia is an electrical problem. Eastern medicine focuses on the meridian system, which is the electrical system of the body. The meridian system has a close relationship with the nervous system, and the nervous system is an electrical system in the body. Acupuncture treatment is designed to work on the body's electrical energy flow. If there are blockages in certain parts of the meridian pathway, the part that is related to the meridian can have a "short circuit," meaning the electrical energy can be interrupted. By stimulating points where blockages occur, acupuncture can unblock the meridian pathway and open the flow of electrical energy.

Acupuncture also helps balance organ energy, including heart energy. Organ energies support each other; for example, spleen energy helps metabolic function and helps govern the blood system. Kidney and liver energy help support heart energy. Lung energy brings more oxygen to the heart and helps maintain dynamic function of the heart and promotes healing.

Tui na therapy for healing is similar to acupuncture. It is a very pleasant treatment and can be very effective if you have a well-trained or experienced practitioner. It relaxes the whole body, opens the energy channels, and soothes the nervous system; patients also benefit from sensing the feel of true care from the special hands-on healing. Often acupuncturists end up getting more patients who prefer tui na therapy. Some acupuncturist use both acupuncture and tui na therapy in treating their patients. Each case is different; some patients need acupuncture, some need tui na therapy, and some can benefit from both.

Qigong or Tai Chi Practice

Qigong can regulate your body organ system and make your body function better. It helps regulate the autonomic nervous system and especially enhances the vagus nerve function, which helps reduce heart rate, relax the muscles of the coronary arteries, reduce blood pressure, and regulate heart rate and rhythm. Therefore, it allows the blood to flow to the heart and other organs. During practice, you can feel your stress reduce right away, and you can feel your heart and mind are at peace. You can feel the healing energy go through your body. Qigong practice helps balance the cardiovascular center in the brain, which also helps regulate heart and blood pressure. The heart benefits of qigong practice are both mechanical and electrical or, you can say, anatomical and energetic.

I studied tai chi in medical school and loved it. I was always curious about qigong because in China there were two different opinions about qigong: some people said it was fake and others said it was real. I have always been a curious person and I like to try to get to the truth.

In 1991, I went to visit my family in Shanghai, China. The day after I landed, I got up early and went to a little open space on the street in Shanghai, not far from my aunt's house. I joined a group of seniors who were doing an exercise routine. In China, people retire at an earlier age, therefore seniors range in age from fifty-five years old to more than a hundred years old.

At the end of the exercise I noticed an older woman with a full head of gray hair. I walked over to speak with this woman and found out she was in her eighties. I asked her why she was doing this exercise in the morning with others. She told me she came here every day, even in the rain. I know doing exercise in the rain is not good for the body, so I asked her why she was so dedicated to this routine. She said she had heart disease for several years. She went to the emergency room several times because of heart attacks. She had to carry medication every place she went, in case of another heart attack. In addition, she experienced fatigue, poor physical strength, and poor digestive function. Her friend recommended this special qigong exercise and suggested she give it a try. After practicing this qigong for a while she felt better overall, felt stronger, was mentally clearer, and she enjoyed doing it. Eventually her heart improved, her energy level improved, and she never went to the emergency room again. I was so interested in hearing this story because I was trained in conventional medicine, which taught me to recommend using either surgery or medication to control the symptoms of heart disease. I was not a believer in the holistic way at that time.

I was so impressed with this woman's story, I decided to learn this qigong exercise from a trained teacher, and then I brought it to the United States. The Chinese name for this qigong is Lian Gong Shi Ba Fa (Practice 18 Methods). I named it Therapeutic Qi Gong. It turns out that this qigong is the most popular form of qigong exercise and has helped many people in physical, mental, and emotional ways.

During my time in Massachusetts (1989 to 2014), I taught this special qigong form in various facilities, such as community centers, senior centers, colleges, companies, and my continuing education program for nurses; to physical therapists and occupational therapists; and in my tai chi school. All of my students loved it, and my patients had good results in their healing. Some patients could not believe how well they felt. They told me that their energy levels improved, their anxiety and stress were reduced, their back pains improved, and their overall joy had returned. I wanted to share this wonderful qigong, and so in 2004, I wrote my first book, *Natural Healing with Qigong*, which was published by YMAA Publication Center.

Qigong should be the first choice for your daily routine if you have heart disease, vascular disease, or hypertension. If you work full time with limited time for qigong exercise, you can still benefit from doing a short qigong form or a portion of this form, multiple times throughout the day—for example when you have a break at work. You will still get benefits from your practice.

For many years, when I worked with patients who had heart disease, I prescribed qigong as their medication, "qi medication." Almost everyone told me that they felt the difference in many ways, in addition to an improvement in their original symptoms.

When I was living and working in Sarasota, Florida, I worked with a man who had heart disease and was recovering from bypass surgery. Unfortunately something happened after surgery, and he had multiple complications and almost died. His nephew found me on the internet and brought him to see me. At the first appointment, he was sad, very depressed, tired, and did not believe anything could help. He was in a wheelchair, pushed by his nephew. After getting to know his medical history, I asked him to do qigong at home. He refused to do the qigong movements I prescribed for him. It got to the point that I shouted at him, "Do you want to die or you want to live?" (I know I should not have shouted at him; I still need to work on my patience!) My intention was to save his health. He replied, "I want to live." That was a good start. I taught him three qigong movements.

In two months, not only did his energy increase, his emotional attitude was amazingly improved. He continues to recover, and his health really took a turn for the better.

Here is part of a letter from his nephew:

When I first visited my uncle in the hospital in October of 2017, not one of his doctors thought he would make anything close to a full recovery. He had gone in for a routine bypass procedure on his heart earlier in the summer of 2017. The bypass itself went quite well, but by October his kidneys had failed, he was on dialysis three times a week, receiving nutrition strictly from a tube and had not been out of bed for five months.

I have studied qigong for the last couple years and as luck would have it, spent some time around some very gifted healers practicing Traditional Chinese Medicine. I found Dr. Kuhn online and after reviewing her website and seeing some of the techniques she shared in her videos I felt grateful to find a practitioner in the area that was the real deal.

My uncle at first refused to meet with Dr. Kuhn. He is an 80-year-old Irishman from NYC and it took some time to break through his preconceived notions about natural healing. Four more months passed by. Not one doctor or nurse thought he had any chance of getting out of his wheelchair. They actually discontinued his therapy a couple times because they thought he had plateaued. Around the new year he had some huge strokes of luck to go along with all the effort he had been putting into therapy and found himself off dialysis and in Feb. off the feeding tube. Though still quite groggy and extreme tiredness, he was more himself than he had been the entire time and I thought it was a good time for him to come home with myself as his caretaker for a transitional period. He came home March 1. Though his internal organs had shown signs of coming back to life his legs were still failing him and one leg could not move. It was at this point that I laid it on really thick and was finally able to convince him to see Dr. Kuhn. In our first meeting he was still grumpy, standoffish and a bit close-minded. His response to Dr. Kuhn asking if he would be willing to do some exercise every day to support the work she would do on him was a very dry "maybe." We still laugh about that one. However, on the way home from that meeting he said to me "You know, she is the first doctor that has ever mentioned me having a chance to walk again." He had one of the moments where the clouds part and the mind opens, his hope restored in the fact that someone else had faith in his potential to heal. That was eight weeks ago. Though he is not running around the house and doing jumping jacks just yet, he is at a point where when I take him to restaurants he does not need a wheelchair at all. He gets along smoothly and safely on a walker. His diet (which was once the diet that lands you a triple bypass) has improved significantly under Dr. Kuhn's guidance. No more bacon for breakfast and red meat all day. He is eating his vegetables and drinking his water. We were able to get his prescription medications reduced by about 75% as well, which has been one of the key points in his recovery to go along with the acupuncture, massage, exercise and dietary regimen that Dr. Kuhn has put him on with great success. He is men-

tally clear, light-hearted and optimistic about his future. Now the grumpy old man who would "never let someone do massage on me" is happy to tell anyone in earshot about his "Natural Chinese Doctor" and the amazing results he has experienced under her care. He is now using walker more and more, doing Qi Gong exercise daily and continues to improve his health. I and my entire family are forever grateful to Dr. Kuhn for sharing her gifts with my Uncle and giving him a new perspective and approach to life based in the power of natural healing!

This is the person who had no clue about qigong and didn't believe natural medicine could help. The good part is that he was willing to try, and just from trying he learned the truth: the body can heal!

I highly recommend that anyone who has heart disease should look into qigong and practice on a regular basis. It will be a life-changing experience. Many people first ask what they can take for their problem; it has always been this way. The truth is, it is not just about what you can take, it is about what you can *do* to change your health and life.

Here is why qigong should be the first choice of exercise for people who have heart disease:

- The movements of Qigong are slow, focused, meditative, and incorporate work with the breath. The practice allows the body to relax and the mind to relax and leads to the opening of the body's energy channels.
- Qigong enhances the function of the vagus nerve system (parasympathetic nervous system), which has a big effect on reducing the heart rate, relaxing blood vessels, relieving stress, and preventing heart disease and hypertension.
- If the qi in the body is strong and balanced, your body and circulation system will be strong and you will be less likely to develop circulatory and vascular diseases. Your qi circulation affects blood circulation, your blood circulation affects qi circulation. There is saying in Eastern medicine: qi is commander of the blood; blood is mother of the qi.

- Qigong brings more oxygen to the body and all organ systems. We all know that oxygen is one of the most important elements in our body that relates to our health and well-being. Oxygen is involved in every metabolic process in our body, and every part of the body needs oxygen to function well.

Your Homework: Practice Qigong

Throughout my years in holistic healing work, I have observed that the best outcomes occur when qigong is incorporated into the treatment plan. It has made an enormous difference in patients' healing.

Qigong is not what some people think it is. It is not mysterious superstition and neither is it "all in your head." Yes, what's in your head is involved. Wanting to feel better and improve your health initiates the action, and from the practice the illness is affected. Very simple. No matter what you believe or do not believe, all that matters is that people feel better, they are happier, and they succeed in their career and life from qi and Dao practice.

Qigong is an ancient Chinese exercise for healing. It has been used for many centuries, and it is getting more and more popular in the modern world. It is used for stress reduction, relaxation, and antiaging. Qigong is an easy form of internal practice. It is easy to learn and practice, which makes it more accessible to more people. The beauty of qigong is that you get results instantaneously; you feel calmer and you have more energy. Qigong is a great antiaging exercise for the brain. It helps clear the mind and improves memory, and that clarity assists in making better life choices. For more information about qigong, please refer to my previous book, *Natural Healing with Qigong.*

Qi refers to vital energy or life-force flow in the body, like the electrical flow in a wire. The various types of qi in the body work together to keep our physical atmosphere in harmony. Qi has a very close relationship to human metabolism, immune function, digestion, absorption, emotions, breathing, and mental clarity. Qi is present internally and externally and controls the function of all parts of the body. Qi is the motor of the body, just like the motor in the car. Qi keeps us moving and functioning, keeps us warm, and protects us against sickness. Everything we do involves qi. Walking, eating, laughing, crying, playing sports, working, hiking, and writing are all related to qi. Qi affects our life every day. We cannot see the qi in the body, but we can feel it. We can feel when our energy is low or when it is high. We can sense if we are optimistic (good qi) or depressed (stagnated qi); we can feel whether our bodies are out of balance (imbalanced qi). From practicing the fundamental qigong that involves mind, body, and breath, one can feel the internal peace, calmness, and strength. Qi is very important in human life.

Many times people tell me they want to get better, but they need to start making changes. If we want to change our health, we must participate in the changes—we need to put our mind into the process of change. I often explain to patients that healing requires two parties to work, both the doctor and the patient. Each party counts for 50 percent of the partnership. If you rely only on your doctor, you get only 50 percent. Therefore you need to put in *your* 50 percent of the effort to make the healing effective. I always give homework to patients who come for a holistic consultation. The people who do their homework show much more improvement than people who do not do their homework. Doing the homework really helps them feel the difference.

Below is the homework for assisting healing or preventing cardiovascular disease and hypertension. If you have family history of cardiovascular disease, start this practice. Practicing three to five times a week is good, but daily practice is highly recommended. During practice, focus on your breath, total relaxation, and how you move your body. You can feel it, connect with it, and embrace it.

Please see chapter 4 for specific instructions on performing qigong exercises to heal or prevent cardiovascular disease.

Mindful Meditation

Mindful meditation is a great practice for assisting in the healing of heart disease. It is a skill that provides a wholesome way to attend to our experiences and helps us overcome the unskillful habits of mind that cause us to suffer needlessly. It is a form of physical and mental exercise that serves to strengthen the natural ability to bring moment-by-moment awareness to our lives. It is nonjudgmental mental and physical practice that involves deep breathing and total relaxation of the entire body. In addition to releasing tension in all muscle groups, mindful meditation helps to de-stress the mind, nourish and cultivate the spirit and qi, restore inner peace, and discover the truth of yourself. The practice of meditation, over time, develops the quality of wisdom and compassion, the virtue of discipline.

Mindful meditation provides great health benefits to our body, mind, and spirit. Some people are negative about meditation and some people love this kind of practice. In the beginning you might find it difficult to stay focused. Many people face this challenge. I suggest you start with a short session of five minutes. Just think a moment and ask yourself, how do I feel in a peaceful environment compared with a busy or stressful environment? The meditation is a process that teaches you to create a peaceful environment for yourself. You can do it anytime, anywhere; all you need is a few minutes. One of the healing aspects of tai chi and qigong is that they are moving meditations, which is a different type of mindful meditation.

At first, practice mindful meditation in a sitting posture, as described below. Later, you can practice standing qigong meditation in what is called the Horse Stance posture. No matter what posture you use, practicing meditation helps remove tension and increase awareness and helps you see things clearly. It also helps you become more nonjudgmental and more focused, which promotes a greater sense of responsibility while maintaining inner harmony.

You don't have to worry about carving a lot of time out of your schedule to meditate. Any time you have can be used for meditation. If you have twenty minutes, that is fine. If you have five minutes, that is fine too. You can practice anytime and anywhere, like in a waiting room or at your desk on your break time. The steps below can be used all together or in any combination of the three.

Practicing meditation is extremely useful in assisting in healing cardiovascular illness and hypertension. People have experienced reductions of blood pressure after five to ten minutes of practice. When your body is totally relaxed, your vascular system is also relaxed, which leads to decreased blood pressure. Heart disease is often caused by chronic stress, and meditation provides a stress-free environment. With diligent practice, your heart starts to heal.

Your Homework: Practice Meditation

Step One: Preparation

Sit quietly and comfortably on a chair or the floor. It is important to be comfortable. Observe the inner activity of your mind—all the mental, physical, spiritual, moral, and ethical aspects. Think about aiming to be a better person and how to become more compassionate. If you had a stressful event before, or the previous day, let it go, because it is in the past. Focus on the present; you can deal with necessary work tomorrow, or after your practice.

Step Two: Focus on Breathing

Start to focus on deep breathing. With each deep inhalation, visualize the abundant oxygen going into your body through your breaths, and pure qi flowing through your body channels and organs. With each exhalation, let go of all anger, fear, hate, grudges, anxiety, and tension. Release anything negative with the exhalation and relax the entire body, letting go of all the tensions in the body: neck, shoulder, arms, upper back, middle back, lower back, hips, knees, ankles, toes. It is easier to focus if you close your eyes. After even a five- to ten-minute practice, you will feel the difference. You will be more relaxed, clear-minded, refreshed, and have a better attitude.

Step Three: Practice Mindfulness

While you are practicing meditation, you put your mind into total relaxation. Relax each muscle group one at time, along with each set of breaths (mentioned above). Your mind must be there the entire time. Pay attention to any tight body part, and intentionally relax it. Try to breathe slowly, and let your mind guide your breaths and control your breaths; focus on how long your breath is, and how deep your breath is. If you are sitting, you can place your hands on your knees with palms facing up. You may feel warmth in the center of your palm after you practice for a while. That is a good thing.

Moving Meditation

I have mentioned before that both tai chi and qigong are called "moving meditation." Moving meditation is a very good practice for people who cannot sit still, or are unable to do sitting meditation. In addition to the benefits of meditation, these exercises provide more health benefits to our body, mind, and spirit. You can find more detailed information about qigong in chapter 4.

Walking Meditation

Many of us walk regularly, but not many practice walking meditation. Walking is good exercise; it offers even more benefits if you add meditation to your walking. Most of us walk with our mind chattering in endless circles. We call this the "monkey mind." If, while you walk, you practice focusing your mind "moment-to-moment," you will feel much more clear-minded, more comfortable in your body, your spirit will be lifted, and you will experience total relaxation.

Here is how to practice:

Choose the path you normally walk, or even just walk in your backyard. As you walk, focus on your breathing, taking deep controlled breaths. Pay attention to what nature provides: trees, the green leaves on the tree; flowers, the shape of the flowers; birds, identify the colors and shapes of the birds; notice the grass, the pond, what you can see in the pond; the river, what is on the riverbank; notice the sky, the colors, the clouds, the shape of the clouds, and so on. Anything from nature is good for you to observe.

Next observe whether you are walking fast or slow; how you are breathing; are you short of breath when you fast walk? Do you hurt anywhere when you walk? How can you adjust your walk, and what is the best type walk for you? Ask yourself, "Am I relaxed?"

During your walk, avoid thinking of other things. This is not easy to do. If your mind wanders, just bring it back to your walk. To get the most benefits from your walk, enjoy the entire experience of your walk. Practice this walking meditation for a few days, then compare it to your regular walk. Can you tell the difference and feel the difference? I feel so incredibly good and energized after my meditation walks. If my mind goes off during my walk, I feel unsettled, and sometimes I feel tired after the walk. Everyone is different, but it doesn't hurt for you to try.

Daoist Learning and Practice

Daoist learning and practice can help you remove life stress. We discussed this in our first book, *True Wellness*. The key to successful practice is your persistent learning and practicing. If you are interested, visit my website for the Tai Chi & Qi Gong Healing Institute (www.taichihealing.org), so you can join our monthly Dao study. It is a life-changing experience.

What Is Dao (Tao)?

The Dao is an ancient Chinese philosophy that is described in the *Dao De Ching*, a book attributed to the writings of Laozi. It explains the principles underlying the universe, and signifies the way or code of behavior that is in harmony with the natural order. The Dao is the natural phenomenon and spontaneous happening that cannot be named or described. Dao is the living wisdom, the methods, and the guide. Dao is the intelligence of human behavior, and the Way.

The *Dao De Ching* emphasizes searching the inner world of perfect self without perfection. Dao helps seekers find true self and inner peace, allowing them to find the inner world, map the beautiful path for themselves. Following the beautiful path, they reach the highest peak and illumination. When that comes, the chaotic world cannot destroy them, or harm them.

Dao is a philosophy, the Way, living wisdom, natural happening, natural phenomenon, non-divided spirit and nature.

Embracing the Dao helped me through every kind of turbulence in my life and kept me from insanity. Dao helped me understand that the perfect self is one without perfection. It is a practice, and I work consistently to improve my weaknesses. It taught me to accept these weaknesses instead of denying them. Through this practice, my life has become easier, happier, and lighter.

Often our minds are too busy. Our thoughts go round and round, seemingly with no purpose, but modern neuroscientists have determined that this constant "chatter" is the brain simply processing information about yourself, your environment, and your memories. This constant state of awareness has been dubbed the default mode network (DMN). This "busy mind" is normal, but can be a distraction during meditation. To calm this busy mind, consider "less" versus "more"; "I need" versus "I want"; "spiritual riches" versus "material riches."

Dao is living wisdom, and it helps everything in life. When you have a relaxed mind, you have a relaxed body and pure spirit. Your health stays balanced. Your relationship tends to be healthy because the Dao is the way to melt and resolve conflict. The Dao brings peace and harmony to your life. Its methods help solve life problems in a gentle way, using humility, modesty, kindness, and forgiveness.

Your Homework: Practice the Dao

Studying the Dao is not difficult, but practicing the Dao is not easy. To study the Dao, you can start by reading one or two chapters of the *Dao De Ching* a day. This 2,500-year-old wisdom/philosophy may not be easy to understand. Take the time to absorb each chapter. Read and reread each chapter. To practice the Dao is to put the theory of its wisdom into your daily practice and awareness. It is a daily mindful practice to be with the Dao. With daily practice it will soon be part of your consciousness. It took me a while to truly understand the essence of Dao and practice it mindfully.

Basic practice

Let go

Letting the past go out of your mind requires daily practice. It is not always easy. In the beginning you may often need to catch yourself and stop your negative thoughts. But after maintaining a mindful practice for a while, it becomes easier. By practicing this, you can move forward and have a better life year after year. If we can let go of unpleasant memories, trauma, anything that is negative, we can move forward with our life. If you are constantly thinking of the past, you are just playing the old tape again and again, and it can hurt you. The past is the past, and there is no need to go back.

Go with the natural flow, not against the flow; yield

Soft overcomes hard. Think of the bamboo yielding to the wind and growing stronger every day. Wisdom comes from learning to go with the flow.

If something stressful is happening in your life, worry and fear do not help you. Consider what actions you can take. In the end we either solve the problem or we let go if we cannot solve the problem. Soft often wins.

Practice simple, less

We are living is a commercial culture and the commercial culture teaches us to want more. But, we don't have to be controlled by commercial culture; we don't have to be like others. We don't have to have what others have. Consider balancing what you want with what you need. Life is too short to stress over wants. Enjoy whatever time you have. Believe it or not, when I have less, I have less stress and enjoy life more. Simplicity is the virtue.

Be humble, observant, and pause; it helps learning

Practice being humble and observant, and pause to learn. Learning stimulates the mind. First learn to make the mind work more efficiently. To make the mind work more efficiently, you must be able to quiet your mind by first learning to empty your mind. Learning to empty your mind comes from meditation with focused smooth deep breathing. Observation skills come from a practice of being observant; this leads to learning. If you talk nonstop, no information can go in, and you will miss some good information from others. Observe without judging. From this practice of being in this quietness, you feel more relaxed. Learning to be humble is a big part of Daoist practice, and it definitely helps you to manage stress and be a better leader.

Nourishing versus fighting

Focus on the word "nourishing" instead of "fighting." Thinking of nourishing a situation creates a positive feeling. For example, we often hear "fighting" cancer. How about we say "healing" cancer? This approach to nourishing our ability to heal instead of fight cancer is leading to some remarkable research. And when you use the words "nourishing, healing, and peace," your energy changes. Use this approach with other diseases; instead of using the word "fighting," think of "healing" heart disease, "healing" arthritis, "healing" your trauma.

True Wellness Approach to Cardiovascular Disease

- **Optimize sleep—at least seven hours of restorative sleep per night.**
- **Reduce stress, increase social connections.**
- **Improve your diet by increasing the amount of plants and decreasing the animal products you eat (DASH diet).**
- **Practice a mind-body therapy twenty minutes each day. Choose whichever activity you enjoy the most from these options: qigong, tai chi, meditation, yoga.**
- **Decrease sodium intake.**

- Eat dark chocolate (at least 70 percent cocoa), but no more than 30 gm/day.
- Drinking red wine, no more than two glasses per day for men or one glass per day for women, may have health benefits. Check with your physician.
- Engage in cardiovascular exercise for thirty minutes most days of the week, and include resistance training.
- Maintain a healthy weight.
- Consider adding CoQ_{10}, fish oil, magnesium, and vitamin D supplements to your diet. Blood tests will be needed to determine the correct dose required to reach normal serum levels.
- Discuss with your physician the addition of hawthorn, 250–500 mg, two to three times/day for hypertension and perhaps prevention of heart failure.
- Continue any medications that you have been prescribed. Do not stop taking your medications until your physician decreases the dose or stops your prescription.

You now have a broad understanding of the causes of heart disease and recommendations to follow in order to heal or prevent these problems. The remaining chapters of this book provide step-by-step instructions and homework to help you develop your own daily healing practice.

CHAPTER 4

Qigong for Healing the Heart and Blood Vessels

THE TERM *QIGONG* is composed of two words. The first, *qi*, has been translated as the "life energy" or "vital force" within the body; *gong* has been translated as "work" or "mastery." Together, the word qigong can be interpreted as "energy work" or the act of mastering one's vital force. Qigong is a healing practice that combines breath control with concentration of the mind. There are many forms of qigong, but they all basically fall within two types: passive or active. Passive qigong is performed seated or lying down and resembles the stances we associate with meditation. This is also known as internal qigong or nei gong. In the active form of qigong, breath control and focused attention are combined with specific movements to create a type of moving meditation. Active qigong, also known as external qigong or wei gong, is similar to tai chi and yoga.

The practice of qigong is an ancient one. These exercises were known by several names over the centuries, including Dao-Yin, "leading and guiding the energy."[1] Earlier in this book we discussed the silk scrolls that were discovered in the Mawangdui tombs in 1973. These silk texts date back to 168 BCE. A chart was found among these scrolls that depicted the Dao-Yin postures. The Dao-Yin Tu (Dao-Yin Illustrations) consists of four rows of eleven postures, forty-four in all. In these illustrations, the roots of most modern qigong practices can be found. There

---

1. Kenneth S. Cohen, *The Way of Qigong: The Art and Science of Chinese Energy Healing* (New York: Ballantine Books, 1997), 13.

were also descriptions of the stances, instructions for the movements, and indications for the use of each exercise. Certain Dao-Yin exercises were deemed valuable in treating low back pain and painful knees; others were indicated for gastrointestinal disorders, and still others were designated to treat anxiety. This demonstrates that not only were Dao-Yin exercises prescribed as a medical therapy, but that ancient physicians appreciated the utility of this type of qigong practice in the treatment of emotional disharmony.[2]

As old as qigong is, its development was likely influenced by the older Indian practice of yoga. The earliest known documentation of yoga was found in the Indus Valley and dates back 5,000 years. Two millennia later, in approximately 1000 BCE, the Upanishads were written. These commentaries emphasize the personal, experiential nature of the journey toward spirituality and elucidate many basic yoga teachings, promoting an understanding of the principles of karma, chakras, meditation, and prana.[3] In India, the vital life force is known as *prana* and pranayama is the cultivation of the life force through breath control. By breathing with intention, the prana is moved through the *nadi* (channels). The intersections of important *nadi* are called chakras. There are many similarities between this system of energy management and that of qigong and Eastern medicine. Qigong requires the same attention and control of the breath and the movement of qi through channels of the body. Interestingly, the locations of many important acupuncture points correspond to the positions of the chakras.

While yoga and tai chi have many benefits, we feel that qigong is the best practice if you are new to these Eastern healing arts, especially if you have any physical limitations that prevent prolonged standing or impede your ability to move between standing and lying positions. Whether you practice nei gong or wei gong, the regulation of the following components are related and inseparable: the body, the breath, the

---

2. Cohen, *Way of Qigong*, 13.

3. Jennie Lee, *True Yoga: Practicing with the Yoga Sutras for Happiness and Spiritual Fulfillment* (Woodbury, MN: Llewellyn Worldwide, 2016), 7.

mind (thoughts), the qi, and the spirit (emotions).[4] The purpose of regulating and strengthening these components is to achieve good health and longevity.

These related and inseparable elements can also be understood, in a traditional sense, as the Three Treasures—*jing, qi,* and *shen.* In Eastern medicine, the Three Treasures are considered the root of life. The *jing* is often translated as essence and, in a Western sense, is akin to your genetic constitution; it is a fundamental substance that is intimately involved with reproduction, growth, and development of the body from birth to death. As we discussed previously, *qi* has been described as the vital, dynamic force that animates the body. It could be considered the current that runs the motor of our metabolism and drives every aspect of our bodily functions. The term *shen* is harder to translate; for our purposes, it can be thought of as our mind or spirit. Depending on the context, the word *shen* can mean immortal, god, spirit, mind, or soul.[5]

By practicing qigong we can strengthen the Three Treasures. Because the *jing, qi,* and *shen* are inseparable, they support and fortify each other, leading to better physical and emotional health and well-being.

It is well beyond the scope of this book to have a complete discussion of the metaphysical aspects of qigong.[6] An in-depth understanding of qigong is not necessary for you to begin your practice. What is necessary? You must focus attention on your breath and be aware of the flow of qi as you move your body with intention.

Qigong is a journey. The goal is not perfection, but incremental improvement in physical, emotional, and spiritual well-being. Patience and persistence is the key to receiving the many benefits of qigong.

---

4. Michael M. Zanoni, *Healing Resonance Qi Gong and Hamanaleo Meditation,* introductory comments, https://docs.wixstatic.com/ugd/9371b9_1f315b1505394b7bb b6ceeb9dc4272a6.pdf.

5. Jwing-Ming Yang, *The Root of Chinese Qigong* (Wolfboro, NH: YMAA Publication Center, 1989), 28.

6. For the interested reader, there are many excellent books on this topic listed in the Recommended Reading and Resources section.

Benefits of Qigong

Qigong practice benefits all parts of the body, including all the organ systems and the brain.[7] In the following section, we discuss some examples of these benefits.

Nervous System Benefits

Qigong offers huge benefits to our nervous systems, both the central nervous system and the peripheral nervous system. Qigong practice helps concentration, improves mental alertness, and helps control emotion. Practice also helps preserve vision and hearing as the body ages.

Cardiovascular Benefits

Qi is dynamic. It performs like a motor that pushes the blood where it should go. If a person's qi is strong and circulates well in the body, their blood will also circulate well. If a person's qi is stagnant or weak, it will cause blood stagnation, which, according to Eastern medical theory, can cause heart disease. Qigong contributes to better heart health by regulating the autonomic nervous system. In particular, these exercises activate the vagus nerve, which is a great way to preserve heart energy, normalize cardiac arrhythmias, and maintain normal blood pressure.

Respiratory Benefits

Through deep and slow breathing, more oxygen goes into the lungs. Slow and deep breathing also activates the parasympathetic (calming) part of the autonomic nervous system. Recall that the nervous system interfaces with the immune system. This process helps the functioning of all cells through proper oxygenation as well as improves defensive energy—which in Western medicine we call the "respiratory immune system"—

---

7. Aihan Kuhn, *True Brain Fitness: Preventing Brain Aging through Body Movement* (Wolfeboro, NH: YMAA Publication Center, 2017), 11.

through modulation of the immune system. The lining of the nose, throat, lungs, gut, and urinary tract all contain immunoglobulin A (IgA). IgA is an antibody in the respiratory tract, which protects it from various germs and pathogens and acts as the first line of defense against bacteria and viruses. If the respiratory immune system is strong, immunoglobulin A can fight germs, making it harder for colds and other respiratory infections to take hold. This is why those who practice qigong generally have fewer illnesses.

Gastrointestinal (GI) Benefits

Qigong can improve stomach and spleen energy, which is related to digestion and absorption. From a Western perspective, qigong regulates the vagus nerve, which also controls digestion. With regular practice, digestive enzymes and digestive movement stay balanced through vagus nerve regulation.

Musculoskeletal Benefits

Once the circulation of the qi and blood are improved, muscles receive more oxygen and blood—the muscles become more resilient, more toned, and stronger. Muscle aging is delayed, and joints become more flexible. Overall, we can maintain a younger body even though we are going through the aging process.

Metabolism and Endocrine System Benefits

Balanced qi also helps balance the body's organ systems, which helps balance metabolism and the endocrine system. Here again, these benefits are due to the effect that qigong has on our nervous systems. The central and peripheral nervous systems are intimately connected to the endocrine and immune systems. Neuroendocrine-immune dysfunction can explain a variety of Western diagnoses, such as chronic fatigue syndrome, also known as myalgic encephalomyelitis.

Immune System Benefits

Qigong helps maintain normal immune function.[8] We have already spoken about how these exercises can improve respiratory immunity and help keep infections at bay. For cancer patients, a healthy immune system can prevent infections during treatment. For those without cancer, a healthy immune system can identify precancerous cells and destroy them.

By balancing the sympathetic and parasympathetic nervous systems, qigong also balances the immune system, so that the immune system is neither too weak nor too strong. A weak immune system will result in recurrent infections. An overly aggressive immune system may result in autoimmune diseases like rheumatoid arthritis. In autoimmune diseases, the immune system turns against the body and attacks normal tissue. Qigong and tai chi help keep the immune system balanced.

Other benefits of qigong include delayed aging, improved balance, reduced risk of falling and injury, and improved memory.[9]

Now it is time to begin your journey and start your qigong practice.

Qigong for Healing and Prevention of Cardiovascular Disease

These qigong exercises were chosen for people who have recovered from a heart attack or heart surgery and who are able to do most normal activities. I (Dr. Kuhn) recommend that you do qigong on a daily basis. Hopefully the exercises will also help prevent future heart attacks and help people avoid heart failure or sudden death.

You will notice that I have given a range for the number of repetitions to do for each movement. The number of repetitions will vary based on your personal energy level, or how well you feel. For example, if you

---

8. Aihan Kuhn, *Simple Chinese Medicine: A Beginner's Guide to Natural Healing and Well-Being* (Wolfeboro, NH: YMAA Publication Center, 2009), 137.

9. For further reading, please see Recommended Reading and Resources at the end of this book.

still have fatigue and are not able to do all of these exercises, you can do just the first few exercise movements. Repeat the movements until you feel you have had enough, before you have a moderate shortness of breath. If you feel fine, do all of the exercise movements.

I have suggested when and how to use your breathing to coordinate the movements. But, remember what is most important: *do not hold your breath.* The coordination of your breath with the movements will improve as you relax and get to know the movements. There is not a perfect way to do the qigong. Just practice.

1. Shake Hands, Arms, and Body

This is a nice light warm-up exercise to start gently stimulating the cardiovascular system.

This exercise helps unblock the meridians (energy channels) in the arms. One of the meridians is the heart meridian. You will need to relax your whole upper body, especially your shoulders.

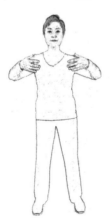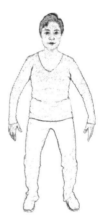

Stand with your feet about shoulder width apart. Bounce gently to shake the body, arms, and hands. Shake your hands from the chest down to your sides in a big motion.

Bounce about 40 to 50 times.

2. Walking and Kicking

Another warm-up exercise. Do this exercise at a pace that is comfortable for you. Your breath should be at a comfortable level.

This movement helps open the meridians in the legs. All the meridians are interconnected and support each other. Therefore all meridians need to be opened to maintain optimum health.

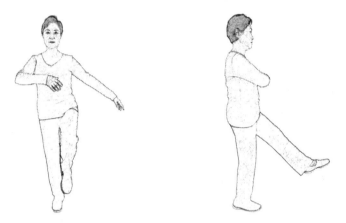

Walk in place. With each in-place step, kick the other leg forward, and swing your arms to the same side.

Alternating sides, do 30 kicks (15 on each side). It will take about 30 seconds.

3. Turn Body Side to Side and Swing Arms

This is also a warm-up exercise.

This movement helps keep the meridian pathways and nervous pathways open.

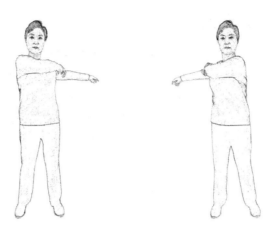

Stand with feet about shoulder width apart. Turn your body from side to side and swing your arms at shoulder level, while keeping your legs straight but not locked. Keep your head facing forward.

4. Open to See the Sky

In this exercise, move slowly and focus on the body movement. Breathe slowly and deeply. Do this exercise and the following ones slowly.

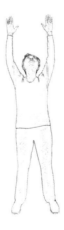

Stand with your feet about shoulder width apart. Take a deep breath. Raise your arms in front of the body until your hands are above your head. Your eyes follow the upward movement of your hands.

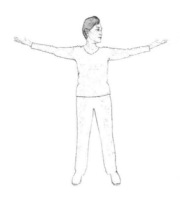

Exhale as you separate your arms, moving them downward to shoulder level. Your eyes follow your left arm.

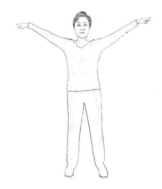

Inhale, turn the palms downward, and raise your arms slightly.

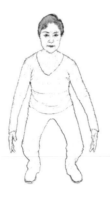

Exhale as you move your arms downward. At the same time, your body sinks.

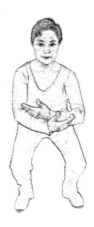
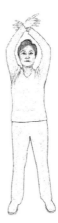

Inhale and return to standing. As you stand, cross your arms in front of your body and raise your hands all the way above your head.

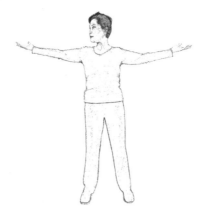

Exhale as you lower your arms to the sides of your body. This time, your eyes follow your right arm.

Repeat this exercise 4 times.

5. Holding Sky Leaning Body

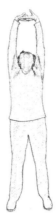

Stand with your feet shoulder width apart. Interlock your fingers and push them up above your head, as you inhale.

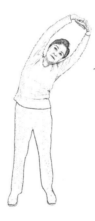

Exhale and lean your body to the left. Stay in this position while you inhale and exhale, completing one breath cycle.

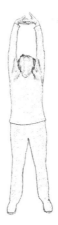

Inhale and return to the upright position, stretching your arms as high as you can, comfortably.

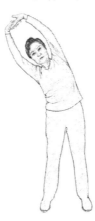

Exhale as you lean your body to the right. Stay in this position for a whole breath.

Repeat this exercise 4 to 8 times. The number of repetitions will depend on how many you feel you can do, comfortably. You should feel stimulated but not overtired.

6. Expand Upper Dan Tian

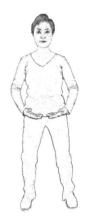

Place your hands in front of your lower abdomen, palms facing upward. The knees are slightly bent.

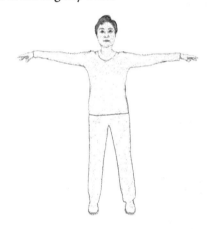

Inhale as you lift/expand your arms to the sides of your body. Open as much as you can. Also lift your heels and straighten your knees.

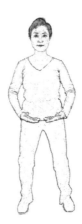

Exhale and lower your heels and unlock your knees. Return your arms and hands to the original position (front of abdomen).

Repeat this exercise 8 times.

7. Horizontal Arm Stretching

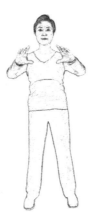

Feet remain shoulder width apart. Place your arms and hands in the front of your body. It will look like you are ready to pass a basketball with both hands.

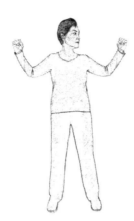

Inhale as you move your arms and hands to your sides while making light fists. Your fists should be about shoulder height. Your eyes follow your left hand.

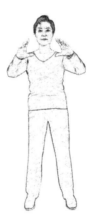

Exhale and move your arms and hands to the front of your body while opening your hands. The arms, shoulders, and hands should be relaxed.

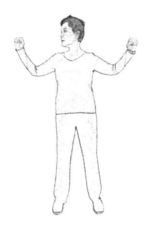

Inhale and move your arms and hands to your sides while making light fists. Your fists should be about shoulder height. This time, your eyes follow your right hand.

Repeat this exercise 8 times (4 times looking left, and 4 times looking right).

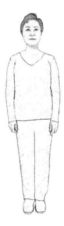

To finish this exercise, exhale as you move your arms and hands down the front of your body and rest them at your sides. Relax your arms, shoulders, and hands, and bring your feet together.

8. Push Up

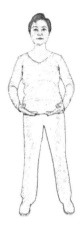

Stand with your feet shoulder width apart. Place both hands in front of your lower abdomen, palms facing up.

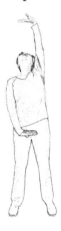

Inhale as you raise your left hand and arm and push it upward, above your head. Push as high as you can. At the same time, your right palm presses downward as low as you can.

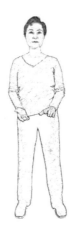

Exhale and move your left hand downward to be level with your right hand, and relax both arms and hands, and the body. Hands are level with your lower abdomen, with right palm facing up and left palm facing down.

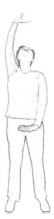

Inhale as you raise your right arm and hand and push it upward, above your head. Push as high as you can. At the same time, your left palm presses downward as low as you can.

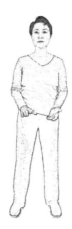

Exhale and relax both arms and hands, also relax your body. Hands are level with your lower abdomen, with the left palm facing up and right palm facing down.

Repeat this exercise 8 times.

9. Qi Go Through Arm Meridians

The heart and pericardium meridians go through your arms. This exercise soothes these meridians.

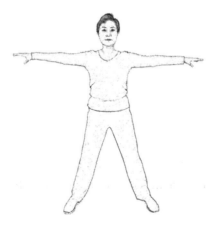

Place your feet so they are wider than shoulder width apart. Inhale and raise your arms to shoulder level, to the sides of your body.

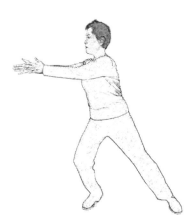

Exhale as you shift your weight to the right leg. Bend your right leg, keeping the left leg straight, but not locked. At the same time, move your left arm toward your right arm. Turn the palms to face each other.

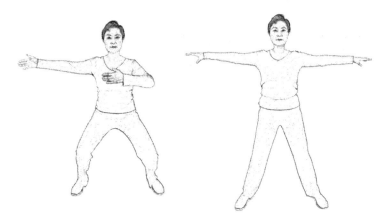

Inhale as you shift your weight back to center, and bend both knees. At the same time, move your left arm across the front of your chest. Continue moving your left arm until it is out to the side. Rotate your palms to face downward. Straighten your legs but do not lock the knees.

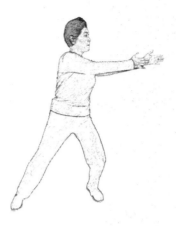

Exhale and shift your weight to the left. Bend your left leg, keeping the right leg straight, but not locked. At the same time, move your right arm toward your left arm. Turn the palms to face each other.

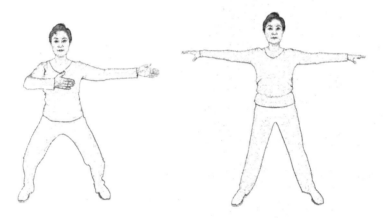

Inhale as you shift your weight back to center, and bend both knees. At the same time, move your right arm across the front of your chest. Continue moving your right arm until it is out to the side. Rotate the palms to face downward.

Repeat this exercise, alternating to the right and left sides, for a total of 4 to 8 repetitions. The number of repetitions depends on how many you can do comfortably.

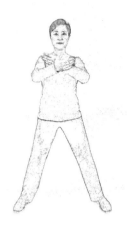
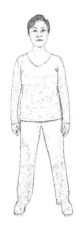

Finish this exercise by crossing your wrists in front of your body. Straighten your legs, then bring your hands and arms down to your sides and relax.

10. Lunge, Turn Body, and Move Arms to Left

For this exercise, adjust your feet as necessary to make yourself comfortable.

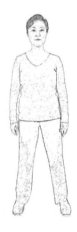

Stand with your feet wider than shoulder width apart.

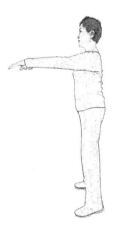

Inhale and raise your arms in front of your body.

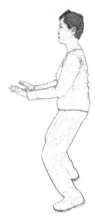

Exhale and sink your body, elbow, and arms.

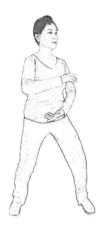

Inhale as you move your arms until they look like they are holding a ball in the front of your body, right hand above left. At the same time, turn your body to the left 45 degrees, and turn your left foot outward 45 degrees.

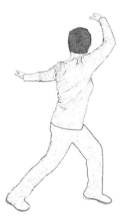

Exhale as you shift your weight to the left leg, turning your left foot (toe) outward 90 degrees or a little more, and turning the right foot (toe) inward about 45 degrees. At the same time, turn your body and move your arms to the left. Your right hand goes above your head and your left arm is at shoulder level.

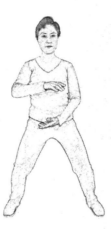

Take a full breath, as you turn your body back to center and bring your arms and hands to the front of your body.

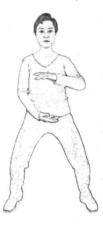

Rotate your hands so your left hand is above your right hand.

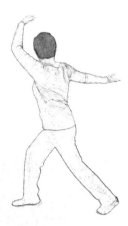

Shift your weight to the right foot while turning your body to the right. At same time, move your arms to the right. Your left hand goes above your head and right arm is at shoulder level.

Repeat this exercise 1 or 2 times.

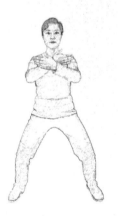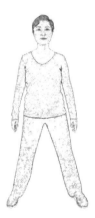

To finish this exercise, return to center and cross your wrists, taking a deep breath. Exhale as you lower your arms to your sides. Take a moment to relax your arms and body.

11. Y Rotation

In this exercise, rotate your upper body slowly and smoothly. Take a full breath (inhale and exhale) with each full circle.

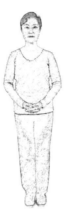

Stand with your feet close together. Interlock your fingers and hold them in front of your lower abdomen.

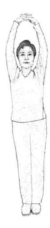

Raise your hands above your head, rotating the palms to face upward.

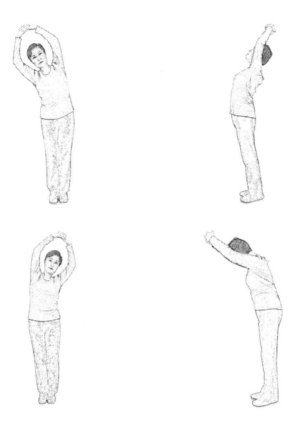

Rotate your upper body to the right, to the back, to the left, then back to the front, so you are making circles with your upper body.

After 4 circles, change direction, and rotate 4 times.

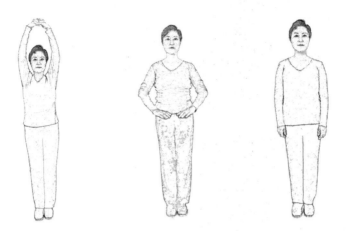

To finish this exercise, bring your body and arms back to center, then slowly move your hands downward. Take a deep breath and relax your body, lowering your arms to your sides.

12. Bending Forward

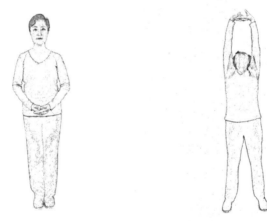

Stand with your feet shoulder width apart. Interlock your fingers in front of your body. Inhale as you raise your arms. Rotate your interlocked hands until the palms face upward.

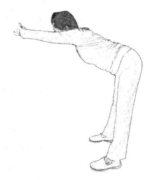

Exhale as you slowly bend your upper body forward and downward. At the same time, move your arms downward.

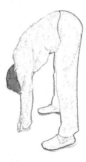

Stay in this position and relax for three deep breaths.

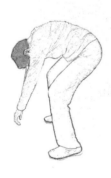

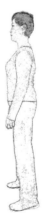

Slowly roll the body back up to standing and relax.

13. Bending Backward

If you cannot hold the positions for one complete breath, you can inhale as you bend backward, exhale, and return to the upright position.

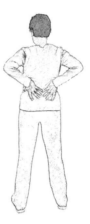

Stand with feet shoulder width apart. Put your hands on your back to support the back.

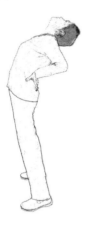 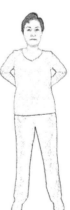

Inhale as you bend the upper body backward and hold this position for one breath. Exhale and return to the original position.

Repeat this movement 1 or 2 times if you are in a weakened condition or have neck or back problems. Repeat 4 to 8 times if you feel comfortable doing so.

14. Knocking the Body

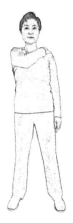 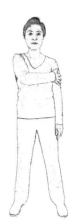

With your right palm or light fist, gently knock on your left shoulder and arm.

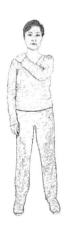 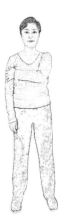

Change sides and, using the left palm or fist, gently knock on your right shoulder and arm.

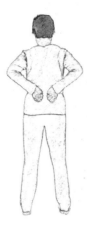

Use both hands or fists and knock on your lower back.

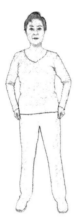

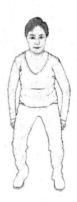

Then, starting with your hip, knock on the lateral part of your legs, moving downward.

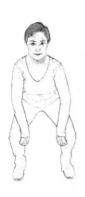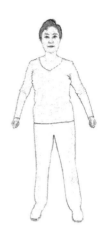

Then knock on the inner part of your legs, moving upward.
Do this for 1 minute.

15. End with Deep Breaths

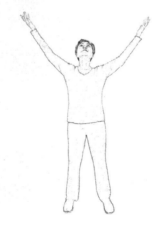

Take a slow deep breath as you raise your arms from the sides of
your body until they are over your head.

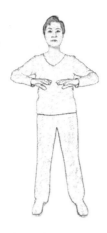 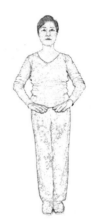

Exhale and move your arms downward in front of your body. The palms slowly press downward.

Do this 3 times.

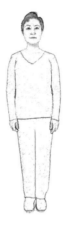

Bring your feet together and relax the entire body.

When you complete this short qigong form, your body will be relaxed, your mind clearer, and your energy will be restored.

CHAPTER 5

The Heart-Mind Connection

THIS CHAPTER IS AN EXCERPT from our first book *True Wellness*. We begin with the first of our Four Steps to Optimal Health—Step One: Build Your Positive Mind. You may be asking yourself, what does the mind have to do with heart disease? Quite a lot, in fact. Recent studies have shown that strong emotions such as hostility, depression, loneliness, and grief are even stronger predictors of coronary artery disease than are smoking and elevated cholesterol. From a biochemical point of view, such emotional states are known to increase IL-6 (interleukin-6), a marker of chronic inflammation. As we have seen, chronic inflammation is instrumental in the development of various types of heart disease.[1]

How to Build Your Positive Mind

A positive state of mind is paramount to your success, allowing you to carry through with any change you wish to make. It is the key to healing on all levels. Practitioners of widely varying systems of medicine, from Eastern to Western, have all noted the same thing: patients who have a positive attitude generally heal faster and remain disease-free much longer than those who do not.

---

1. Mimi Guarneri, *The Heart Speaks: A Cardiologist Reveals the Secret Language of Healing* (New York: Simon and Schuster/Touchstone, loc. 788, Kindle version), 2006.

Our mind is a very special entity. It has tremendous power and can contribute both positively and negatively to our health. If used to create positive changes, the mind can help heal many illnesses, whether psychological, physical, or spiritual.

Changing the mind can change behavior; changing behavior can change health, relationships, and life circumstances.

A positive mind makes positive physical changes: relaxed muscles, reduced heart rate and blood pressure, balanced metabolism and blood sugar, and improved production of digestive enzymes. A negative mind produces negative physical results: tight muscles, irregular or fast heart rate, elevated blood pressure and blood sugar, low energy, poor metabolism, decreased enzyme production, and difficulty sleeping.

Some of these negative physical states had a purpose in the past. It would have been an advantage to have elevated heart rate, blood pressure, and blood sugar when running from a predator or combating a foe. This physical state, caused by the release of stress hormones such as adrenaline and cortisol, is known as the fight-or-flight response. It was instrumental to our survival as a species, but in modern-day life we often do not allow ourselves to recover from these extreme episodes. We subject ourselves to many daily stressors, strive to meet sometimes unrealistic expectations, and often fail to nourish our bodies and minds. Physiologically, we are forever preparing for the next battle, just as our ancestors were; however, the constant secretion of these stress hormones can be detrimental to the body and the mind.

Your mind not only affects these physical elements but also influences the social, behavioral, and interpersonal aspects of your life. It goes without saying that most people prefer the company of positive individuals. A positive mind involves love. Positive individuals often exude love. Love brings joy, healing, and happiness. Giving love and receiving love both arise from a positive state of mind. Love does not have conditions or bias. Love involves giving, selflessness, compassion, and kindness. Love produces healing results through a sense of inner peace. You love your family and your friends, but it is the love and compassion you give to yourself that will make the difference in your healing journey. It will allow you to develop a positive mind and lead a healthy life by quieting the fight-or-flight response and decreasing the release of stress hormones.

A positive mind that is calm and compassionate can help control emotions and cravings. This is why some people are better able to manage stress and achieve their objectives. A positive mind can improve your mental ability, concentration, and determination; however, other aspects are involved in reaching your goal.

Every completed action, such as altering habits, is predicated on making a decision to change and then actually carrying out that decision. A person's ability to follow through on resolutions can be influenced by many things. Although many emotional components are involved, successfully making profound behavioral changes is not a matter of willpower alone.

From a Western perspective, making lifestyle changes requires not only desire and determination but also healthy brain chemistry. The compounds that convey messages throughout your brain and body are called neurotransmitters. Neurotransmitters are influenced by many factors, such as sleep patterns, exercise, nutrition, and meditative practices like qigong and tai chi.

Dopamine is the neurotransmitter that is released when you perform any action that results in a feeling of accomplishment. Any such pleasurable activity increases the secretion of dopamine. You can use this reaction to your advantage when trying to reinforce behavioral changes. Every time you complete a questionnaire or exercise in this book, reward yourself. The reward could be large or small. It may help if the reward reinforces the behavior you are trying to reinforce; for example, downloading great new music for your workout or purchasing a fancy kitchen gadget to prepare new, healthy recipes.

The purpose of the reward is to increase dopamine release. Then you will want to take the next step in your transformation. Pamper yourself with larger rewards for each accomplishment. If you never find time to read, curl up with a good book. If you love to paint, enroll in an art class. Play sports with friends, treat yourself to a movie, or purchase a new item of clothing. All these sorts of activities will release dopamine, and you will want to continue on your healing path. Every time you reward yourself for performing a positive behavior, you will strengthen the association between that behavior and a feeling of well-being. You will reinforce positive, healthier habits.

Western neuroscientists have observed that positive reinforcement actually changes the way your brain functions. Using special magnetic resonance imaging studies called functional MRIs, researchers have shown that people who practice this technique increase the number and activity of neural connections in various parts of the brain. They are, in fact, changing their minds. This property of the brain is called neuroplasticity, and results from studying it are altering the way conventional medicine looks at the brain, from both the physiological and psychological point of view.[2]

From an Eastern perspective, successfully making changes is a matter of common sense. Food, rest, activity, and self-reflection must be balanced to lead a healthy life. In today's hectic world, we may need some reminders about how to build a positive mind to achieve physical, emotional, and spiritual equilibrium. To this end, we have created a series of home study activities for building a positive mind.

The mind and body are intricately intertwined. Any variation in one aspect will cause changes in the other. This is why building a positive mind will have such an important effect on your body. The question is, what can you do to alter internal processes on such a deep level? There are three interconnected ways to approach this task:

- Change the way you *breathe*.
- Change the way you *think*.
- Change the way you *act*.

The following pages are full of written exercises to guide you through this transformation. While some space is provided for short answers, we

---

2. Norman Doidge, *The Brain That Changes Itself* (New York: Viking/Penguin, 2007), 11.

recommend you start a journal for daily entries. Your journal can be electronic or on paper. Remember to give yourself an appropriate reward for completing these homework assignments, which will reinforce your new behaviors, encourage persistence, and lead you to a state of true wellness.

Breathe

You may have noticed that some of the calmest, most centered individuals are those who engage in an activity that involves slow, deep breathing. These may be yoga practitioners, tai chi or qigong enthusiasts, or those who regularly meditate; maybe they only follow the habit of taking three deep breaths whenever they are upset. But the link between a tranquil demeanor and deep breathing is no coincidence: there is a direct connection between how breathing patterns are interpreted by the brain and the resulting emotion that a pattern will evoke.

Give this a try:

Start breathing very shallowly and rapidly for ten to twenty seconds. (Stop if you start to feel faint!) Notice how you feel, emotionally. Agitated? Anxious? Fearful? Describe your sensations here:

_____

_____

_____

Now take three long, deep breaths. How do you feel? Most people will say they feel calmer, more peaceful, or more relaxed. Write down your experience here:

_____

_____

_____

This association between breathing patterns and emotion has been demonstrated by a number of researchers, including Pierre Philippot. Philippot conducted an interesting pair of studies in which he showed that specific emotions evoke particular breathing patterns that usually occur when someone exhibits that sentiment. This pattern was consistent from person to person. He went on to show that the reverse is also true: when test subjects were asked to breathe in a particular pattern, they reliably stated that they experienced the associated characteristic emotion.[3]

Regulation of the breath is a part of many medical traditions and has been used for millennia to calm the mind and heal the body. From Tibetan meditation to the modern "relaxation response," from yoga to tai chi and qigong, the breathing techniques incorporated into these modalities can balance the sympathetic and parasympathetic nervous system through the modulation of neurotransmitters released in the body.[4]

Homework

Choose an activity that causes you to breathe in a pattern that allows you to feel both calm and alert. This could be qigong, tai chi, yoga, or meditation. It could be some other activity of your choosing. Pay attention to your emotions during these slow, deep breaths. It is OK if your attention wanders, as long as you keep coming back to your breath. Perform this activity for five to ten minutes each day, longer if desired.

Every day that you complete this homework, give yourself an appropriate reward. After several weeks, you will find that you won't need this reinforcement as often, if at all.

---

3. "Respiratory Feedback in the Generation of Emotion," http://www.scribd.com/doc/164856193/Respiratory-Feedback-in-the-Generation-of-Emotion-Philippot-2013, accessed December 25, 2013.

4. T. M. Srinivasan, "Pranayama and Brain Correlates," *Ancient Science of Life* 11 (1/2): 1–6; D. Krishnakumar, M. R. Hamblin, and S. Lakshmanan, "Meditation and Yoga Can Modulate Brain Mechanisms That Affect Behavior and Anxiety," *Ancient Science of Life* 2 (1): 13–19, doi:10.14259/as.v@i2il1.171; Michael M. Zanoni, "Healing Resonance Qi Gong and Hamanaleo Meditation," https://www.mikezanoni.com/meditation-qi-gong, accessed February 4, 2018.

Think

Thoughts and emotions are two different things. Although they are inextricably linked, they are not the same. An emotion does not arise spontaneously. It is felt in response to a thought. It is not possible to change an evoked emotion, but it is possible to change the way you think.

So, how do you go about changing your thoughts? You challenge them. Take a step back and examine your thoughts about yourself and the world around you. Often our thoughts produce negative emotions such as fear and self-criticism. But is what you think really true? Are you exaggerating your situation, if only slightly? If your thoughts are true, then what? For example, say you are giving a big presentation at work. You know it is important. You might even get a promotion if you do well. You worry that if you botch it, your boss and coworkers will think less of you. You might even make yourself anxious thinking about it. But take a moment and challenge these thoughts. If your employee or coworker is giving a presentation and stumbles, do you think she is an awful person? Would you fire her? If you are working in an environment where this could be true, then consider how it is affecting your life and your physical and emotional health. It is certainly reasonable to acknowledge your nervousness before entering into a stressful situation such as public speaking, but with practice you can stop that emotion from generating a downward spiral of negative thoughts.

Use Your Fear

Fear is a double-edged sword. It can be a powerful motivator or a destructive force. Fear of blindness caused by diabetes can prompt you to control your blood sugars. Fear of a stroke might make you exercise and meditate to lower your blood pressure. However, fear that immobilizes you is debilitating: it stops you from acting to prevent that which you fear. This in turn makes you more fearful. Being stuck in this vicious, unproductive cycle generates many negative physiological responses in the body and mind. You are forever in the fight-or-flight response, in a constant state of stress.

What would happen if you let this unproductive fear go? It is not easy to have a fear-free life, but it can be achieved through practicing mindfulness. Preparing answers and actions for things that could happen helps remove fear: preparing for the worst thing that could happen can help you be less fearful and less stressed. Through your actions, you may be able to avoid negative experiences, but if something really happens, you will know how to deal with the situation.

Homework

Ask yourself these questions and write down your answers:

What do I fear?

_____

_____

_____

_____

How likely is it that the things I fear will come true?

_____

_____

_____

_____

What steps can I take to prevent this from happening?

_____

_____

_____

_____

What steps will I take to improve my situation if these fears come true?

_____

_____

_____

_____

_____

Look for Solutions Instead of Complaining

It is human nature to complain. It is easy to get into a rut, complaining about a situation without making an effort to change it. Sometimes we have issues or problems from various life experiences. Instead of complaining, which can negatively affect ourselves and others, we need to try to find solutions.

Life is not always easy; that is part of learning. You learn to solve problems through adversity. Every time you find an answer or solve a problem, you feel a sense of achievement; you feel ready to take on the next challenge that lies ahead.

If you can look at a problem without fear, without attachment to the outcome, a solution will often present itself. The solution may not be complete—it may only be a step in the right direction—but it will alter the nature of your circumstances. You may think such a tiny shift is too insignificant to matter, but it is the accumulated momentum of individual small actions that creates the process of change.

Homework

Think of a personal problem that has been unresolved for a long time. Now think of the outcome you desire. Write down one or more ways that you could solve this predicament. At this point, there is no need to act on your ideas. Consider as many creative solutions as possible and write them down here:

_____

_____

_____

_____

Find Something Positive in Everything

When you come across something negative, ask yourself, "What is positive in this situation?" Changing the way you think and looking for the positive aspects of a situation can improve your energy. When you look on the positive side of things, you allow yourself to heal. People who are always looking at the negative side of a situation can build a barrier to their healing path.

One of my (Dr. Kuhn's) patients cured her chronic headaches simply by changing her viewpoint from negative to positive. For many years, "Heather" had ongoing headaches that affected her life and made her fatigued all the time. When she started to see me, Heather mentioned that she had a lot of stress from both work and home. At work, she was a manager of forty people in a big corporation. She felt overwhelmed all the time and sometimes had to make difficult decisions. At home, her husband cared for their two young children, and Heather felt guilty because she was less involved in child care than she wanted to be.

Regarding her work-related stress, I asked, "Do you do the best you can at work?" Heather said yes. I explained to her that she should be satisfied with what she has done for the company because that is all she can do. Since she did the best she could, there was no need to feel stressed. Regarding Heather's home stress, I asked her, "Are your children and husband happy at home without you present?" She replied, "Yes, they are very happy." I explained to her that since they were happy, then she should be happy, not stressed. The breadwinner has to work to provide the others with comfort and necessities. Heather was making herself ill by thinking of things in a negative way. Soon after she understood this and saw the positive side of her situation, Heather's headaches were greatly relieved and were almost all gone within several days. As Heather continued to view her situation in a positive light, her headaches resolved, her energy improved, and she became happy both at work and at home.

Homework

It is not easy to be positive all the time, but it can be achieved by daily mindful practice. Whenever you have a negative experience, write down one positive aspect of that encounter below. For example, you are given a task at work that involves learning new procedures. It may take more time and effort at the beginning, but eventually you have mastered a new skill that you can add to your résumé.

_____

_____

_____

_____

_____

_____

Be Thankful

Many cultures around the world devote certain holidays or special occasions to giving thanks for whatever comforts they have in life. Some years these comforts may be few, but there is always something for which to be grateful. Appreciation and gratefulness are a part of many religions. A sense of thankfulness to some higher power, something outside ourselves, can change our outlook for the better.

It really does not matter if you are religious. It is not about organized religion; it is about spirituality. Having a belief system that incorporates regular expressions of gratitude has many healing benefits. Various researchers have documented the positive effects of articulating appreciation.

R. A. Emmons and M. E. McCullough demonstrated that members of a study group who, on a daily basis, wrote in a journal about things, people, or situations for which they were grateful noted superior life improvements than did those in groups assigned to chronicle their problems or how they were better off than others. The life improvements noted in members of the grateful group included increased "alertness, enthusiasm, determination, attentiveness, and energy." They also reported being able to exercise longer, sleep more deeply, and stay asleep for greater periods of time.[5]

The above benefits were not simply the subjective impressions of the study participants. When friends, family members, and colleagues were asked to describe grateful individuals, such individuals were more likely to be rated as happier, helpful, optimistic, and trustworthy.[6]

Expressing appreciation and gratitude decreases the release of stress hormones and increases hormones such as serotonin, which balance your nervous system. You will feel calmer, more optimistic, and more motivated. With this kind of reinforcement, you can move forward with ease.

Homework

Every day for the next month, write down one thing that you appreciate or for which you are thankful. You will likely need to use your journal, but just to get you started, write down three experiences for which you are grateful:

_____

_____

_____

Always Have Tomorrow

We all feel down or unwell from time to time. Tell yourself, "Tomorrow I will feel better." It is true; the next day is different. We all have ups and

5. R. A. Emmons and M. E. McCullough, "Counting Blessings versus Burdens: Experimental Studies of Gratitude and Subjective Well-Being in Daily Life," *Journal of Personality and Social Psychology* 84 (2003): 377–389.

6. M. E. McCullough, R. A. Emmons, and J. Tsang, "The Grateful Disposition: A Conceptual and Empirical Topography," *Journal of Personality and Social Psychology* 82 (2002): 112–127.

downs, rainy days and sunny days. We sometimes feel overwhelmed, frustrated, and have bad experiences. If we keep thinking about these negative feelings, we can feel stuck with these pessimistic moments. Our energy can be depleted. If we tell ourselves, "Tomorrow will be a better day" or "Things will change tomorrow," we don't feel as frustrated, and we feel calmer instead.

Our brain gets rest overnight. Often our troubles seem smaller in the morning. Daily meditation also calms the brain and allows you to approach a problem refreshed and clear-headed. Being able to take a step back, whether for a ten-minute pause to meditate or a full night's sleep, allows you to see things in a more positive light.

Act

Now that you are changing the way you breathe and think, it is time to act. There are three actions you can take to build your positive mind:

1. Forgive

2. Reach out

3. Change your dynamics

Forgive

The first and most important action is to forgive. The first and most important person to forgive is yourself. We all have regrets and imperfections, but everyone can improve and make changes. If you can forgive yourself, you can forgive others. This is a type of mindfulness practice that can be incorporated into, and assisted by, regular meditation.

If you don't forgive, you are holding on to negative energy, and the negative energy can make you sick. Forgiving can assist healing and is also part of healing. Forgiveness can be toward anyone or everyone. Forgiving is not the same as excusing, condoning, or forgetting wrongful behavior. It is possible to forgive someone for morally "unforgivable" acts. If you choose to forgive someone who has harmed you, that person's underlying behavior or character may not change. By choosing to forgive, you are changing the relationship dynamics and taking steps to end the control that person has over your well-being. Practicing forgiveness can eliminate resentment and be a powerful motivation for people to move forward, be happy, and heal.

Various studies over the last decade have shown that the act of forgiving can have positive health benefits, both physical and emotional. These include lower blood pressure, lower risk of alcoholism or substance abuse, less anxiety, and better relationships with others.[7]

By being compassionate, forgiving yourself and others, you can bring balance to the part of your nervous system that controls the fight-or-flight response. Self-compassion has even been associated with decreased inflammation and protects against inflammatory and autoimmune diseases.[8]

While doing the following forgiveness exercises,[9] you would do well to remember the famous words of St. Augustine: "Resentment is like taking poison and hoping the other person dies."

Homework

1. If you feel you have been wronged or have hurt another person, think about whether the situation has affected your physical, mental, or spiritual health. Describe these symptoms here:

_____

_____

_____

---

7. Mayo Clinic, "Forgiveness: Letting Go of Grudges and Bitterness," http://www .mayoclinic.com/health/forgiveness/MH00131, accessed December 25, 2013.

8. J. G. Breines et al., "Self-Compassion as a Predictor of Interleukin-6 Response to Acute Psychosocial Stress," *Brain, Behavior, and Immunity* 37:109–114. pii:S0889-1591(13)00537-0, doi:10.1016/j.bbi.2013.11.006.

9. Mayo Clinic, "Forgiveness: Letting Go of Grudges and Bitterness," https:// www.mayoclinic.org/healthy-lifestyle/adult-health/in-depth/forgiveness/art -20047692?pg=2, accessed January 6, 2018.

_____

_____

2. Choose to forgive or ask forgiveness from the person or people involved. If it is not possible to speak directly with these individuals, write a journal entry or note (which you may or may not decide to send). In one or two sentences, without accusation or excuse, give or ask for forgiveness here:

_____

_____

_____

_____

_____

3. Understand that this process may take time. As you forgive others or receive forgiveness, notice how your physical, mental, or spiritual state has changed. List these transformations here:

_____

_____

_____

_____

4. If you are having difficulty letting go of resentment or grudges, you may want to seek the help of an unbiased friend or relative, spiritual counselor, or medical professional. List at least three trusted individuals here and arrange a meeting as soon as possible.

_____

_____

_____

_____

Reach Out

Many people are afraid to reach out, but developing social connections and a sense of community can have many benefits. By reaching out, you learn from others: you get positive energy and support. You also have the opportunity to contribute to your social network, which will increase your own feelings of belonging and self-worth.

By seeking out social relationships, you may even increase your life expectancy. Researchers at Brigham Young University performed a meta-analysis of 148 studies, involving more than three hundred thousand people. This study showed that, over a seven-year period, having social relationships decreased the risk of dying by 50 percent. It did not make a difference whether you had a preexisting medical condition, whether you were male or female, or even whether you were young or old; stronger social relationships predicted a longer life.[10]

To put it another way, the health risk inherent in low social interaction is equivalent to other well-known health risks such as smoking fifteen cigarettes a day or being an alcoholic. Being socially isolated is more harmful than not exercising and twice as harmful as being obese.

Reaching out to others will not only help you build a positive mind, but will also help extend your life!

Homework

1. At least once a week, contact an old friend or talk to a colleague about something other than work. List these contacts here:

_____

_____

_____

_____

10. Julianne Holt-Lunstad, Timothy B. Smith, and J. Bradley Layton, "Social Relationships and Mortality Risk: A Meta-Analytic Review," July 27, 2010, http://www.plosmedicine.org/article/info:doi/10.1371/journal.pmed.1000316#s4.

2. Every week, schedule a social engagement with a close friend or casual acquaintance. It could be as long as a day at the beach or as short as quick coffee after work. List these outings here:

_____

_____

_____

_____

3. Join an organization of people with whom you share a common interest. For example, if you play a musical instrument, join a community orchestra. If you enjoy sports, join a local league. If you like ethnic food, take a cooking class. Write down six group activities and do the one you would enjoy the most.

_____

_____

_____

_____

4. Volunteer your time at a community institution of your choice, like the Humane Society, a food bank, or your public library. Write down six organizations in your area and offer your help to the one that interests you most.

_____

_____

_____

_____

Change Your Dynamics

You can change your dynamics, both internally and externally. So far, the homework you have done is helping you change your internal dynamics and build your positive mind. An important attribute of a positive mind is an open mind. When you keep an open mind, you are more likely to try new experiences and meet new people. Every new encounter will stimulate your brain and make changing your old routines much easier.

Let's look at a common situation: many people do not like their jobs. They feel like they have to do their job just to pay the bills. That is not healthy; saying "I hate my job" will decrease your energy. If, instead of saying "I hate my job," you say, "I learn from this job no matter what," your energy changes. This will change the energy of the working environment, and you may find amazing results.

For example, say hi to every single person you meet at work. If you are usually disorganized, then make a plan for each workday. If you micromanage your colleagues, call a brainstorming meeting about an issue that needs to be solved, and let your colleagues run with their ideas. Buy a cup of coffee for a person you usually hesitate to talk to; invite a coworker to lunch, or take a walk together. You may not hate your job anymore once you are more open-minded, willing to try new approaches, and have changed the energy in your work situation.

Now push yourself to change your dynamics outside of work. Take a different route home. Sample new foods. Pick a radio station at random and listen to it for a while. All these shifts in your routine cause your brain to stop running on autopilot and pay attention to your inner and outer environment. When you are truly aware of what is going on around you, your brain creates new neural pathways. By changing how you act, you can change the way you think; you are more likely to feel inspired, energized, and ready to meet life's challenges.

Homework

1. Write down your daily routine here:

_____

_____

_____

_____

2. Every day for the next week, pick one item from the list above and substitute an alternative action. List the old/new pair each day and describe any difference you notice in your thoughts or feelings at the end of the day.

_____

_____

_____

_____

Even though you have reached the end of step one, remember we are never fully finished building our positive mind. You may want to revisit some or all of these pages during your journey toward true wellness as a reminder to breathe, think, and act with compassion, optimism, and gratitude.

CHAPTER 6

General Principles of Self-Healing

ULTIMATELY, THE SUCCESSFUL TREATMENT of cardiovascular disease, in fact all disease, depends on consistent self-care. Even if you are taking medications for these conditions, you must be attentive to your body, mind, and spirit on a daily basis. Medications must be taken regularly without skipping doses, and doctors' appointments should be kept. There is a lot that your health-care provider can do, from arriving at a correct diagnosis to arranging specialty and support services.

But there is even more that you can do for yourself. We all know that eating nutritious foods, not smoking, exercising regularly, sleeping adequately, and managing stress levels can lead to a healthier life. In fact, the World Health Organization (WHO) and Centers for Disease Control (CDC) have determined that by exercising more, eating better, and not smoking, 40 percent of cancers and 80 percent of adult-onset diabetes and heart disease could be prevented.[1] Sleep deprivation and life stress have each been shown to contribute to the incidence of chronic illness, so sleeping well and managing your stress can decrease your risk for such diseases.

Taking care of yourself requires determination. Every day you will be faced with choices about what foods to buy, how to cook them, how

---

1. Kenneth Thorpe and Jonathan Lever, "Prevention: The Answer to Curbing Chronically High Health Care Costs (Guest Opinion)," May 24, 2011, http://www.kaiserhealthnews.org/Columns/2011/May/052411thorpelever.aspx.

much to eat and how to exercise and for how long. You also make choices about whether to go to sleep at a reasonable hour or stay up and surf the internet. You choose whether to manage your stress by meditative practices or dangerous habits such as smoking or excessive alcohol consumption. Every decision you make matters. Your doctor can give you advice, but ultimately, you must decide for yourself and act on those decisions. No one else can do it for you.

If you have already established these healthy habits, congratulations! You are stacking the odds in your favor. The likelihood that you will develop a lifestyle-related chronic illness is at least half what it would be otherwise. As we have seen, even conditions like heart disease can be improved through lifestyle modification.

If you feel there is room for improvement in the way you eat, exercise, and manage your stress, now is the time to gear up and get going. In our first book, *True Wellness: How to Combine the Best of Western and Eastern Medicine for Optimal Health*, we devoted a whole chapter to the process of change, setting goals, and taking action to achieve those objectives. We have found that one of the most useful tools you can use to establish new habits is a checklist. There is nothing particularly glamorous or high-tech about a checklist, but for many people, it is invaluable. With a checklist, you can see concretely what you have or have not done during the course of your week. If you plan to practice qigong three times a week, you can see as the days pass whether you will meet that goal. If you are honest, you will see the number of times you meditated or went to the gym, how many vegetables you ate, or how much water you drank. Many people, when they start using a checklist, are astonished at their own lapses. We often convince ourselves that we are doing all we can to achieve optimal health, when really we are falling short of the mark. This sort of wishful thinking is very common.

The beauty of a checklist is that it gives you a systematic way of changing your behavior and developing consistency. The checklist has become integral in air-traffic safety procedures and in hospital operating rooms. Its use has improved outcomes in these industries where lives hang in the balance. It is not being too melodramatic to say that both the quality and quantity of your years on Earth depend on establishing habits that maximize your physical, emotional, and spiritual health.

Decades of medical research show that most chronic illnesses are lifestyle driven and that the underlying physiological problem in these conditions is chronic inflammation. Many studies demonstrate that eating a minimally processed plant-based diet; meditating; practicing qigong, tai chi, or yoga; exercising regularly; and getting adequate sleep all decrease chronic inflammation. Using the True Wellness Checklist can effectively support your shift toward healthy lifestyle, decrease chronic inflammation, and reduce your risk of developing many chronic conditions.

The True Wellness Checklist

Instructions for Use

The True Wellness Checklist is a compilation of recommended actions that are associated with optimal health. These actions form the basis of disease prevention in both Eastern and Western medical systems. Meditation, qigong, cardiovascular exercise, and resistance training should be incorporated into everyone's healing plan. Optimizing your sleep can improve your physical and emotional health. Sleep has an enormous effect on all chronic conditions. This is why we have included in this custom version of the True Wellness Checklist measures you can take to improve the quality and quantity of your sleep.

Many people have food sensitivities, allergies, or individual preferences; therefore, the dietary recommendations on the checklist form the essentials of a vegan regimen. You can add servings of meat, fish, and/or dairy, depending on your tastes or requirements. The majority of your food should be plant-based. If you do eat animal products, your plate should be filled three-quarters with plants and only one-quarter with animal protein. Choose whole foods over processed foods. Minimize sweets, but on occasion enjoy chocolate made of at least 70 percent cacao.

Approximate serving sizes

Vegetables	1 cup raw vegetables, ½ cup cooked vegetables
Fruit	1 medium piece of raw fruit, ½ cup canned fruit, ¼ cup dried fruit
Nuts	⅓ cup
Beans/Legumes	½ cup cooked
Whole Grains	1 slice of bread, ½ cup cooked grains, 1 ounce dry cereal
Red Meat, Poultry	cooked, roughly the same size as a deck of cards
Fish	uncooked, 8 ounces (no more than 3x/week because of heavy metals)
Dairy	1 cup of yogurt, 1 cup of milk, 2 ounces of cheese
Eggs	1 egg
Oils	extra virgin olive oil (cooking/dressings), flaxseed oil (dressings)

True Wellness Checklist

Daily Practice	Day 1	Day 2	Day 3	Day 4	Day 5	Day 6	Day 7
sleep							
• Wake up at the same time every day	☐	☐	☐	☐	☐	☐	☐
• Meditate daily	☐	☐	☐	☐	☐	☐	☐
• No caffeine after 3:00 p.m.	☐	☐	☐	☐	☐	☐	☐
• No naps after 3:00 p.m.	☐	☐	☐	☐	☐	☐	☐
• Exercise no later than 3 hours before bed	☐	☐	☐	☐	☐	☐	☐
• No electronics 1–2 hours before bed	☐	☐	☐	☐	☐	☐	☐
• Keep bedroom cool and dark	☐	☐	☐	☐	☐	☐	☐
• Go to bed at the same time every night, if sleepy	☐	☐	☐	☐	☐	☐	☐
• If not asleep in 15 minutes, engage in relaxing activity without electronics, then lie down again when sleepy*	☐	☐	☐	☐	☐	☐	☐
food							
• Vegetables (4–6 servings daily)	☐	☐	☐	☐	☐	☐	☐
• Fruit (3–4 servings daily)	☐	☐	☐	☐	☐	☐	☐
• Nuts (1/3 cup daily)	☐	☐	☐	☐	☐	☐	☐
• Beans/Legumes (1–2 servings daily)	☐	☐	☐	☐	☐	☐	☐
• Grains (3–4 servings daily)	☐	☐	☐	☐	☐	☐	☐
• Water (8 glasses daily)	☐	☐	☐	☐	☐	☐	☐
• Protein of choice	☐	☐	☐	☐	☐	☐	☐
move-ment							
• Cardiovascular exercise (2–5x/week)	☐	☐	☐	☐	☐	☐	☐
• Resistance training (2–5x/week)	☐	☐	☐	☐	☐	☐	☐
• Qigong or Tai Chi (5–7x/week)	☐	☐	☐	☐	☐	☐	☐
fun							
• At least one 15-minute activity every day, simply for your own enjoyment	☐	☐	☐	☐	☐	☐	☐

*Suggested activities: read a book (an old-fashioned hard copy), meditate, do restorative stretching or qigong, have a warm bath or shower, listen to calming music, breathe in a pattern where your exhalation is about twice as long as your inhalation.

Conclusion

SCIENTIFIC THOUGHT IS ALWAYS EVOLVING. During the last half of the twentieth century, researchers in biology, chemistry, mathematics, and physics realized that sometimes understanding individual components of system was not sufficient for understanding the system as a whole. They developed different ways of thinking about the multiple causes and effects that affected the networks they studied. With these observations came the realization that the whole system is greater than the sum of its component parts. This understanding is the foundation of Eastern medicine and is the antithesis of reductionist Western medical thought. Happily, the field of conventional medicine is changing its philosophy and is also adopting this whole-systems-based approach.

Our purpose in writing *True Wellness for Your Heart* is to help our readers view their cardiac difficulties differently: not as isolated medical conditions, but as problems within the whole system. It is not enough to simply take a pill to treat high blood pressure or undergo bypass surgery to allow blood to flow around a blocked coronary artery. You must look at all the underlying causes in the genesis of any disease. Treating the symptoms alone will not remedy the imbalance in the system that allowed the illness to emerge. Without correcting the underlying issue, the imbalance will worsen in spite of medical treatment or manifest in another part of the body.

To easily visualize this concept, let's use a boating analogy. Let's say that you are sailing along when suddenly you notice that you are knee-deep in water. Immediately, you start bailing water out of the boat. You may even have pumps that automate this process. Even if you can bail as fast as the water is coming in, there will be consequences to the flood over time; the electronics will start to short out, mold will start to grow. Your boat may not sink immediately, but it will be ruined nonetheless, if you can't find the breach in the hull.

Until recently, for complex chronic conditions like heart disease, Western medicine has been bailing water. For too long, our population has been getting sicker and sicker, in spite of targeted medications and surgeries. Finally, though, our attention is turning to the breach in the hull. Conventional medical practitioners are looking at the whole system, treating patients as whole people with their unique environments and relationships. Together they are learning that the best way to get to the root of the cardiovascular disease may be examining the quality of a person's sleep, nutrition, meditative practices, and social connections.

Eastern medicine has always been rooted in whole-systems philosophy, so integrating this modality into conventional cardiac care further enhances the holistic approach that some Western practitioners are taking. We hope that you will use this book as a guide toward more robust health in all respects: body, mind, and spirit.

Acknowledgments

W E WOULD LIKE TO TAKE THIS OPPORTUNITY to thank all our advisors, reviewers, illustrators, and editors, who keep the momentum going as we continue on with the "True Wellness" series. At YMAA Publication Center we are appreciative of the efforts of publisher David Ripianzi and editor Leslie Takao, whose knowledge of the Dao and qigong was invaluable. Production manager Tim Comrie, illustrator and designer Axie Breen, and publicist Barbara Langley have all been enormously helpful. At Westchester Publishing Services, we would like to thank director of editorial services Susan Baker and copyeditor Susan Campbell for polishing the manuscript.

We are indebted to Dr. Bart Denys for his advice and improvements to the body of the manuscript. Dr. Denys's qualifications as a cardiologist and an acupuncturist give him a unique perspective on the integration of Eastern and Western medicine in the treatment of cardiovascular disease, and we are grateful that he brought these insights to light in writing the foreword for this book.

Recommended Reading and Resources

Websites

American Academy of Medical Acupuncture, https://www.medicalacupuncture.org/Find-an-Acupuncturist

American College of Cardiology, "CardioSmart," https://www.cardiosmart.org

American Heart Association, https://www.heart.org

Centers for Disease Control and Prevention, "Heart Disease," https://www.cdc.gov/heartdisease/index.htm

National Certification Commission for Acupuncture and Oriental Medicine, https://www.nccaom.org/find-a-practitioner-directory

National Institutes of Health, DASH Diet Guide, https://www.nhlbi.nih.gov/files/docs/public/heart/dash_brief.pdf

National Institutes of Health, US National Library of Medicine, Medline Plus, https://medlineplus.gov/howtopreventheartdisease.html

Tai Chi & Qi Gong Healing Institute, www.taichihealing.org

Books

Chatterjee, Rangan. *How to Make Disease Disappear.* New York: HarperCollins, 2018.

Chatterjee, Rangan. *The Stress Solution: The 4 Steps to Reset Your Body, Mind, Relationships, and Purpose.* London: Penguin Life, 2018.

Chinnaiyan, Kavitha. *The Heart of Wellness: Bridging Western and Eastern Medicine to Transform Your Relationship with Habits, Lifestyle, and Health.* Woodbury, MN: Llewellyn, 2018.

Cohen, Kenneth. *The Way of Qigong: The Art and Science of Chinese Energy Healing.* New York: Ballantine Books, 1997.

Doidge, Norman. *The Brain That Changes Itself.* New York: Viking/Penguin, 2007.

Doidge, Norman. *The Brain's Way of Healing.* New York: Penguin, 2015.

Guarneri, Mimi. *The Heart Speaks: A Cardiologist Reveals the Secret Language of Healing.* New York: Atria, 2010.

Harris, Dan. *10% Happier: How I Tamed the Voice in My Head, Reduced Stress without Losing My Edge, and Found Self-Help That Actually Works—A True Story.* New York: HarperCollins, 2014.

Helms, Joseph. *Getting to Know You: A Physician Explains How Acupuncture Helps You Be the Best You*. Berkeley, CA: M.A.P. Medical Acupuncture Publishers, 2007.

Jauhar, Sandeep. *Heart: A History*. New York: Farrar, Straus, and Giroux, 2018.

Jonas, Wayne. *How Healing Works: Get Well and Stay Well Using Your Hidden Power to Heal*. New York: Penguin Random House, 2018.

Kaptchuk, Ted. *The Web That Has No Weaver: Understanding Chinese Medicine*. New York: McGraw-Hill, 2000.

Keown, Daniel. *The Spark in the Machine: How the Science of Acupuncture Explains the Mysteries of Western Medicine*. London: Singing Dragon, 2014.

Kuhn, Aihan. *Natural Healing with Qigong: Therapeutic Qigong*. Wolfeboro: YMAA Publication Center, 2004.

Kuhn, Aihan. *Simple Chinese Medicine: A Beginner's Guide to Natural Healing and Well-Being*. Wolfeboro, NH: YMAA Publication Center, 2009.

Kuhn, Aihan. *Tai Chi in 10 Weeks: Beginner's Guide: A Proven Step-by-Step Plan for Integrating the Physical and Psychological Benefits of Tai Chi into Your Life*. Wolfeboro, NH: YMAA Publication Center, 2017.

Kurosu, Catherine, and Aihan Kuhn. *True Wellness: How to Combine the Best of Western and Eastern Medicine for Optimal Health*. Wolfeboro, NH: YMAA Publication Center, 2018.

Lee, Jennie. *Breathing Love: Meditation in Action*. Woodbury, MN: Llewellyn Worldwide, 2018.

Lee, Jennie. *True Yoga: Practicing with the Yoga Sutras for Happiness and Spiritual Fulfillment*. Woodbury, MN: Llewellyn Worldwide, 2016.

Oz, Mehmet. *Healing from the Heart: A Leading Surgeon Combines Eastern and Western Traditions to Create the Medicine of the Future*. New York: Plume, Penguin, 1998.

Scheid, Volker, and Hugh MacPherson, editors. *Integrating East Asian Medicine into Contemporary Health Care*. Edinburgh: Churchill Livingstone/Elsevier, 2012.

Walker, Matthew. *Why We Sleep: Unlocking the Power of Sleep and Dreams*. New York: Scribner, 2017.

Weil, Andrew. *You Can't Afford to Get Sick: Your Guide to Optimum Health and Health Care*. New York: Plume, 2009.

Yang, Jwing-Ming. *The Root of Chinese Qigong: Secrets for Health, Longevity and Enlightenment*. 2nd ed. Wolfeboro, NH: YMAA Publication Center, 1989.

Glossary

acupuncture. A system of medicine that involves inserting fine metal needles into specific anatomic locations to treat a variety of illnesses and conditions. Derived from the Latin *acus* (needle) and puncture.

American Academy of Medical Acupuncture (AAMA). A society, founded in 1987, of medical doctors (MDs) and osteopaths (DOs) who have undergone training in acupuncture in order to incorporate this modality into conventional health care.

American Board of Medical Acupuncture (ABMA). An independent entity within the AAMA, established in 2000, to conduct examinations of candidates seeking certification in medical acupuncture in order to maintain high standards for the profession.

American Medical Association (AMA). A professional association of medical doctors (MDs) and osteopaths (DOs) founded in 1847. The stated mission of the AMA is to "promote the art and science of medicine and the betterment of public health."

artery. Type of blood vessel that conducts blood away from the heart.

Ben Cao Gang Mu (Compendium of Materia Medica). An encyclopedic medical volume detailing the herbs and other substances used in Eastern medicine. Written in the sixteenth century CE by Li Shi-Zhen, a prominent physician in the Ming dynasty.

blood pressure. The pressure exerted on blood vessel walls by the force of blood moving through the vessels.

blood vessels. Tubular conduits of varying size and thickness through which the pumping action of the heart circulates blood, oxygen, nutrients, and waste products to and from the cells of the body. Types of blood vessels include arteries, capillaries, and veins, which are connected in sequence from arteries to smaller arteries, called arterioles, to capillaries, then to small veins called venules, then to the veins; see artery, capillary, vein.

Buddhism. A philosophical practice that developed out of the teachings of Siddhartha Gautama in the fifth century BCE, from northeastern India through Asia and globally. Gautama became known as Buddha and taught that life is full of suffering, but that suffering could be overcome by developing wisdom, integrity, and awareness.

capillary. The smallest type of blood vessel, only one cell layer thick, where the exchange occurs between oxygen and nutrients in the blood and carbon dioxide and waste products in the cells of the body.

cardiac. Relating to the heart.

cardiac arrhythmia. Any abnormal rhythm of the heartbeat.

cardiovascular disease. Disease involving the heart and blood vessels. Also known as heart disease.

cardiovascular system. Organ system made up of the heart and blood vessels that circulates blood cells, oxygen, and nutrients to the cells of the body. Also circulates blood to the lungs for oxygenation and removal of carbon dioxide and moves other waste products of cellular metabolism to the liver and kidneys for processing and removal; see circulatory system.

circulatory system. Organ system made up of the heart and blood vessels that circulates blood cells, oxygen, and nutrients to the cells of the body. Also circulates blood to the lungs for oxygenation and removal of carbon dioxide and moves other waste products of cellular metabolism to the liver and kidneys for processing and removal; see cardiovascular system.

Confucianism. The teachings of Confucius, which emphasize correct behavior in the institutions and individuals within society as well as the cultivation of knowledge and good judgment.

Confucius. Chinese philosopher, political figure, and educator who lived during the fifth and sixth centuries BCE, whose teachings are known as Confucianism.

coronary artery. An artery that supplies oxygenated blood and nourishment to the heart.

coronary artery disease. Disease of the coronary artery caused by inflamed, cholesterol-filled plaques that narrow the caliber of the artery and decrease oxygenated blood flow to the heart muscle.

Dao De Ching. A Chinese text regarding the philosophy of Daoism, attributed to Laozi (see Daoism), which may actually be a compilation of works by later authors.

Daoism. Also known as Taoism. The doctrine of living in harmony with the natural order of the universe, ascribed to the teachings of Laozi, a Chinese philosopher who lived during the sixth century BCE.

Eastern medicine. A system of medicine that arose in Asia that makes use of herbal remedies, acupuncture, meditation, qigong, and tai chi to improve health. Also known as East Asian medicine or Oriental medicine.

Five Phases. The cosmological scheme that describes interactions among natural phenomena, such as the changing of the seasons, developed in ancient China millennia ago and used in astrology, military strategy, and medicine. Also referred to as the Five Elements; see Wu Xing.

functional magnetic resonance imaging (fMRI). An imaging technique that employs magnetic and radio waves, used to determine which areas of the brain are most active at the time of the imaging.

gene. A sequence of DNA that codes for a molecule that has a specific function within a living organism; see DNA.

heart. Muscular organ of the cardiovascular system that contracts rhythmically, pumping blood, oxygen, and nutrients to all cells of the body via the blood vessels.

heart disease. Disease involving the heart and blood vessels. Also known as cardiovascular disease.

heart valve. Thickened leaflets of tissue located between the atria and ventricles and between the ventricles and pulmonary artery and aorta that are pushed open by the force of blood moving in the correct direction. Between heartbeats, the valves close to prevent backflow of blood.

Huang Di Nei Jing (The Yellow Emperor's Classic of Internal Medicine). An ancient Chinese medical text written approximately during the Han dynasty (206 BCE–220 CE).

Hua Tuo. Famed second-century CE Chinese physician and surgeon who also developed longevity exercises called Five Animal Qigong.

hypertension. Blood pressure that is higher than normal; see blood pressure.

hypotension. Blood pressure that is lower than normal; see blood pressure.

integrative medicine. A branch of conventional Western medicine that is patient-centered and incorporates techniques from other medical systems for which there is good evidence of safety and efficacy.

Journal of the American Medical Association (JAMA). A peer-reviewed medical journal published by the AMA containing research papers, reviews, and editorials that relate to the field of medicine.

Laozi. A Chinese philosopher who lived during the sixth century BCE and developed the doctrine of living in harmony with the natural order of the universe, a doctrine known as Daoism or Taoism.

licensed acupuncturist (LAc). Designation given to a person who has received a license to practice acupuncture from a state medical or professional licensing board. To qualify, that person must have completed a specific amount of training and passed certifying examinations in acupuncture and Eastern medicine

mind-body medicine. A group of therapeutic practices that engage the mind's capacity to influence bodily functions; examples of these techniques include meditation, relaxation, biofeedback, and hypnosis.

myocardial infarction. Also known as a heart attack, the damage caused to the heart muscle by insufficient flow of oxygenated blood through the coronary arteries; see coronary artery.

National Certification Commission for Acupuncture and Oriental Medicine (NCCAOM). A nonprofit organization established in 1982 to certify competency of acupuncturists, herbologists, and bodyworkers of Eastern medical disciplines in the United States. The NCCAOM is also involved with recertification, examination development, and continuing education for practitioners.

neuroplasticity. The ability of the brain to form new connections and pathways in response to learning or training; also known as brain plasticity.

placebo. A substance or intervention that has no active ingredient or expected benefit.

placebo effect. A positive, unexpected benefit seen following administration of a placebo. Attributed to the recipient's expectation of benefit, considered a mind-body interaction that activates the recipient's innate ability to heal.

post-heaven qi. Eastern medicine term for energy (qi) extracted by the body from food and air.

pre-heaven qi. Eastern medicine term for energy (qi) that is inherited from our parents, analogous to genetic constitution in Western medicine.

preventive medicine. A medical specialty that focuses on the prevention of disease, not only in the individual patient but also in the community and population at large. A combination of clinical medicine and public health.

PubMed. A free search engine that can be used to find abstracts and articles on life sciences and biomedical subjects, maintained by the National Center for Biotechnology Information at the US National Library of Medicine.

pulmonary. Relating to the lungs.

qi. Eastern medicine term for the intelligent life force that flows through the body, often described in Western terms as "energy."

qigong. Mental, physical, and breathing exercises that cultivate qi. Related to tai chi; see tai chi.

Silk Road. Ancient trading route between Asia and Europe that traversed Korea, China, India, Persia, and Europe.

Sun Si-Miao. Prolific seventh-century CE Chinese physician and herbalist who wrote two thirty-volume works on the practice of medicine. He was renowned for integrating Daoism with Buddhism and Confucianism and emphasized ethical behavior for physicians.

tai chi. A Chinese martial art form, but also a series of slow, meditative movements that, when performed regularly, can improve health and well-being. Related to qigong; see qigong.

tui na. A method of Chinese bodywork or massage.

vein. Type of blood vessel that conducts blood toward the heart.

World Health Organization (WHO). An agency of the United Nations, established in 1948, intended to improve international public health.

Wu Xing. Known in English as the Five Phases or Five Elements. The cosmological scheme that describes interactions among natural phenomena such as the changing of the seasons, developed in ancient China millennia ago and used in astrology, military strategy, and medicine.

yin-yang theory. The theory that states that all phenomena are composed of two opposite conditions or characteristics. These opposites cannot be separated; together, they represent the unified whole.

Index

About the Authors

Dr. Catherine Kurosu

Born, raised, and trained in Canada, Dr. Catherine Kurosu graduated from the University of Toronto School of Medicine in 1990. She completed her internship and residency at the same institution and qualified as a specialist in obstetrics and gynecology in 1995. Dr. Kurosu has studied and worked in Canada, the United States, Mexico, and Chile. Through her travels, she has learned that there are many ways to approach a problem and that the patient usually understands their illness best. By combining the patient's insight with medical guidance, effective treatment plans can be developed.

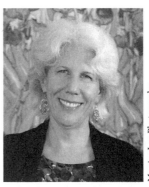

Monica Lau Photography

In 2006, Dr. Kurosu became a diplomate of the American Board of Holistic Medicine, now known as the American Board of Integrative Holistic Medicine. In 2009, she became certified as a medical acupuncturist through the David Geffen School of Medicine at UCLA and the Helms Medical Institute. Dr. Kurosu became a member of the American Academy of Medical Acupuncture, then a diplomate of the American Board of Medical Acupuncture, which confers this title to practitioners with increasing experience.

Since then, Dr. Kurosu has completed a master of science in Oriental medicine, graduating from the Institute of Clinical Acupuncture and Oriental Medicine in Honolulu. In 2015, she became a licensed acupuncturist and in 2018 a diplomate in Oriental medicine through the National Certification Commission for Acupuncture and Oriental Medicine.

Dr. Kurosu now lives on Oʻahu with her husband, Rob, and daughter, Hannah, where she practices integrative medicine, blending Western and Eastern approaches to patient care.

Dr. Aihan Kuhn

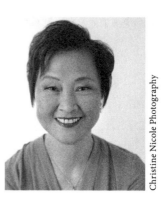

A graduate of Hunan Medical University in China (now called Xiangya Medical School) in 1982, Dr. Aihan Kuhn has oriented her focus to holistic healing since 1992. During many years of practice, she has accumulated much experience with holistic medicine and achieved a great reputation for her patient care and education work. Her patients benefit from her many important tips for self-improvement in their physical, emotional, and spiritual well-being, as well as simple and easy healing exercises to enable them to participate in healing. Dr. Kuhn incorporates tai chi and qigong into her healing methodologies, changing the lives of those who have struggled for many years with no relief from conventional medicine. Dr. Kuhn provides many wellness programs, natural healing workshops, and professional training programs, such as tai chi instructor training certification courses, qigong instructor training certification courses, and wellness tui na therapy certification courses. These highly rated programs have produced many quality teachers and therapists. Dr. Kuhn is president of the Tai Chi & Qi Gong Healing Institute (www.taichihealing.org), a nonprofit organization that promotes natural healing and prevention.

Dr. Kuhn lives with her husband, Gerry Kuhn, in Sarasota, Florida. For more information, please visit her website at www.draihankuhn.com.

Christine Nicole Photography

BOOKS FROM YMAA

DVDS FROM YMAA

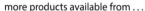

more products available from . . .

YMAA Publication Center, Inc. 楊氏東方文化出版中心

1-800-669-8892 • info@ymaa.com • www.ymaa.com